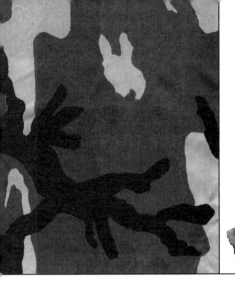
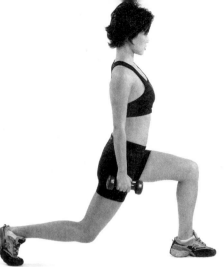
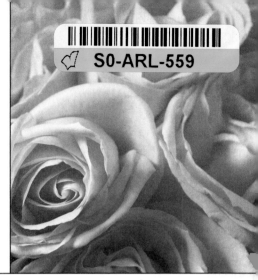

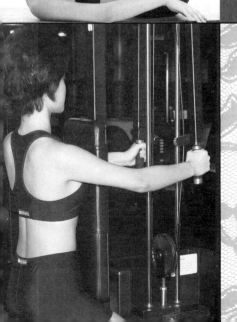

Bridal BOOTCAMP™

by Cynthia M. Conde

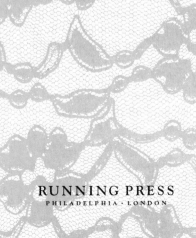

RUNNING PRESS
PHILADELPHIA · LONDON

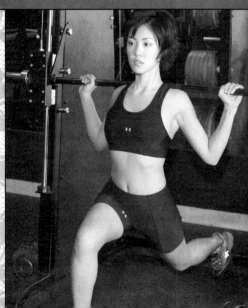

9   8   7   6   5   4   3   2
Digit on the right indicates the number of this printing

Library of Congress Control Number: 2002038214

ISBN 0-7624-1818-4

Cover and interior design by Corinda Cook
Exercise photography by Gilbert King
Model: Shirley Xu
Make-up artist: Mary Anne Mendes
Edited by Deborah Grandinetti
Typography: Galliard, Avenir, Sloop Script, and Stencil

Photographs © by Gilbert King except:
Author photo on back cover, © Jori Klein
Front cover (top left & top right), back cover (bottom right), pp. 1 (top right), 10 (top right & bottom center), and 168 (top left): © Stockbyte/ PictureQuest
Front cover (bottom left), p. 168 (bottom center): © BananaStock/ BananaStock, Ltd./ PictureQuest
pp. 21, 27, 30, 31, 37: © Corbis Images
p. 168 (bottom right): © PhotoDisc/ PictureQuest

This book may be ordered by mail from the publisher. Please include $2.50 for postage and handling.
But try your bookstore first!

Running Press Book Publishers
125 South Twenty-second Street
Philadelphia, Pennsylvania 19103-4399

Visit us on the web!
www.runningpress.com

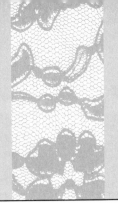

Dedication

To my best friend, Richard Hartmann. Thanks for your loyalty, trust, and patience.

To my mother and father, Awilda and Fernando Conde. Thank you for everything.

To Pandora Kinard. The eighty pounds you lost in time for your upcoming wedding inspired me to create the Bridal Bootcamp™ Fitness System.

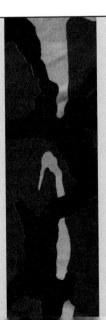

Contents

Introduction 7

PART I: BASIC TRAINING

Before You Enlist 11

The Hardcore Nutrition Program 15

The Bridal Bootcamp™ Supplement Program 38

Fitness Maneuvers: Learning the Exercises 44

PART II: BOOTCAMP!

Six Months to the Wedding 169

    What to Eat 170

    The Workout 191

Three Months to the Wedding 204

    What to Eat 205

    The Workout 225

One Month to the Wedding 236

    What to Eat 237

    The Workout 257

Conclusion 266

Index 268

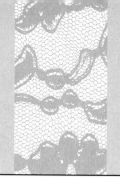

Acknowledgements

Special thanks to my client, Don Imus. His gracious exposure allowed me to write this book.

I also would like to thank my agent, Sheree Bykofsky, and Denise Macwan of IoCandy, for her amazing website and graphic design. Dr. Ken Leistner greatly assisted me with both his time and kindness. I am grateful to Pamela Liflander for helping me gather my thoughts on paper, to Gilbert King for his skillful photography, and to Shirley Xu, our beautiful model, for being so patient and doing a great job. Thanks also to Deborah Grandinetti for editing this book and making this project run so smoothly. Last, I would like to thank to Carlo DeVito, the associate publisher at Running Press, for making this book happen.

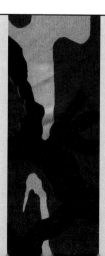

Introduction

The pressure is off, or has it just begun? You've met the man of your dreams, and I bet he loves you just the way you are. But every woman knows that a wedding is more than just two people proclaiming their undying love: it's probably one of the few opportunities you'll ever have to wear a fabulous dress and parade in front of your friends and family without being laughed at. You bet you want to look good!

With *Bridal Bootcamp™,* your success is assured. Do you want great looking arms and shoulders? You'll have them. Do you want the energy to dance all night? You'll have it. Do you want to drop a dress size or more, or to flatten your stomach for a more flattering fit? With this program, you can lose a pound or two per week.

The meal plan and workout routines I provide in this book will get you into the best shape of your life.

I'm confident of your success because I have made the program work for others. I am a certified personal trainer and nutrition consultant who has taught countless clients how to get in shape and maintain a healthy lifestyle. I created the *Bridal Bootcamp™* program years ago when I helped a client lose more than eighty pounds for her wedding. Now it's your turn.

The program works because it is a complete system, one that integrates nutrition with strength training, stretching, and cardiovascular conditioning. You won't get the same results from just dieting alone, or just from exercise. I know—I've tried every trendy diet in the past ten years, and found that just dieting doesn't work. Just exercising doesn't cut it either. So what's the answer? You already know: you have to eat smart and work out.

Bridal Bootcamp™ makes doing both easier for you by taking away the guesswork. It provides specific meal plans and specific workouts, designed to tone every part of your body. If you want to work out at home, I will show you how to get the same results you could get in a gym, using minimal home equipment. If you belong to a gym, I'll tell you which machines to use, in which order, to get maximum results.

Bridal Bootcamp™ also respects your time. You can complete each workout in an hour. On some days, you'll only need to work out for twenty minutes. If your figure is not in the shape you want it to be, now is the time to do something about it. Don't wait until the week before the wedding to begin your dozen-grapefruits-a-day diet. If you have inches to lose and muscles to tighten, you need to allow adequate time to take the pounds off and make sure they don't come flying back. That's why the book features a Six Months to the Wedding nutrition and fitness program, a Three Months to the Wedding nutrition and fitness program, and a more intensive One Month to the Wedding nutrition and fitness program.

To get the results you want, commit yourself to each part of the program. You'll need to follow the guidelines for:

Proper nutrition: The eating plan is both calorie-conscious and nutritious. You'll learn to eat the foods—in the right portion sizes—that will help you lose weight. Better yet, you will lose fat, not muscle, at a pace that is safe for your body and easier to maintain. Also, the foods I recommend are both satisfying and delicious. By following the program, you will not feel deprived, starved, or worse, annoyed. This program is a lifestyle change: a new way of eating that will allow you to have control over your weight forever.

Proper supplements: It is nearly impossible to get the right nutritional balance even when you aren't trying to slim down. Vitamin and mineral supplements are necessary in order to meet your body's requirements without adding calories. These supplements will also supply the additional energy you'll need for the Bootcamp exercise program.

Strength training: You want to increase lean muscle mass, which will in turn shape and tighten your body. Weight training focuses on the areas of the body that you want to tighten up in order to look great in your wedding dress: arms, shoulders, chest, back, legs, and abdomen.

Cardiovascular conditioning: The most efficient way to get rid of excess fat is to burn it. The best way to burn fat is during aerobic exercise. My program is based on an adapting interval cycle, which means your body will continue to burn calories while you increase your workload. Ultimately, your body will become leaner, meaner, and healthier.

Think of me as your personal drill sergeant. I'll be there every step of the way, coaching you through the rigors of the program. My tips will help you stay the course and get the results you desire.

If you follow my lead, I promise the results will be extraordinary. You will look fit and feel confident on your big day. And you will also learn how to eat, exercise, and care for your body so you continue to look and feel great for the rest of your married life.

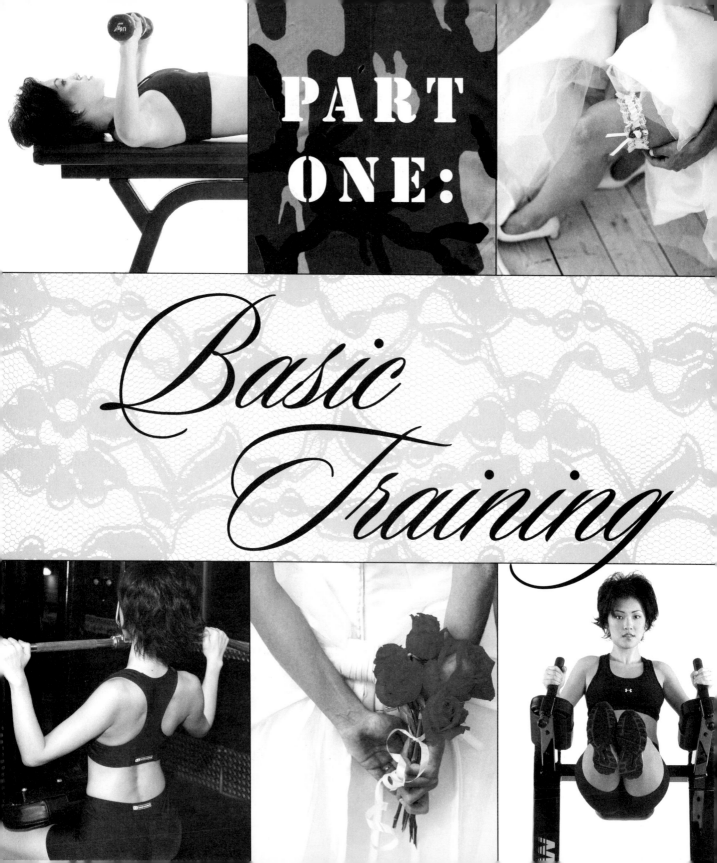

PART ONE:

Basic Training

CHAPTER ONE:

Before You Enlist

Before you start this or any other exercise and diet program, make sure to get your doctor's OK. This fitness boot camp is challenging. If you do have a health condition or an injury, your doctor may suggest dietary or training modifications that will better suit your needs.

I also recommend that you get a chiropractic examination. A good chiropractor can determine if you have any postural alignment problems that might lead to debilitating injuries. A chiropractor can also identify individual joint or nerve problems, and weak muscles. This is invaluable information, and will give you confidence that you can achieve your fitness goals injury free.

Once you've seen your doctors, decide whether you intend to work out at home, at the gym, or both. If you exercise at home, you'll need to pick up some equipment from the sporting goods store immediately. Here's what you'll need:

- Exercise or yoga mat
- In-line skates or traditional bicycle
- Physioball (exercise ball)
- Free weights: 5, 10, and 15 pounds
- Jump rope

If you'd rather use the gym workouts I provide, make sure your gym has the following equipment:

- Stair climber
- Treadmill

- Elliptical climber
- Recumbent bike
- Large selection of strength training machinery
- Dumbbells
- Medicine ball
- Physioball

Whether you work out at home or the gym, you will also need the following:

Exercise shoes: Twenty-first century technology has improved almost every aspect of our lives, down to our shoes. Today, an average-priced running shoe will provide all the support you will need for any type of workout. Choose a cross training shoe if you do not intend to run or walk as your primary aerobic exercise.

Exercise clothing: True exercise clothing is designed not only to look good, but to be highly functional. Try to choose pieces that are soft to the touch, including all openings, seams, and linings: soft materials will prevent chafing. While cotton used to be the preferred choice, today's high-tech fabrics wick away the moisture from your body to the clothing's outer surfaces, so you feel significantly drier throughout your workout.

Sports bras: It is imperative that you wear a sports bra during exercise, whether you are an A-cup or a DD-cup. There are basically three types to choose from. The first are compression bras that press the breasts toward the chest and limit movement. They are recommended for small to medium-breasted women. For large-breasted women, encapsulation bras surround and support the breasts with reinforced seams and wires. Combination bras offer the best features of the other two varieties.

Heart rate monitor: This is by far the most important piece of exercise equipment that you will ever purchase. A heart rate monitor is exactly what the name implies: it records your heart rate during various states of exercise so that you can see how productive you are. The monitor straps onto your torso, just below the chest, and is connected to a wrist-band so you can easily view your heart rate. When purchasing a heart rate monitor, look for a model that will display not only the heart rate, but your percentage heart rate. I recommend the Polar @3 because it displays your average heart rate, your maximum heart rate—which is the method that we use to determine if you are in the right training zone—

and your exercise duration. It also automatically determines your age-based heart rate target zone, allows you to set an alarm, and displays the time and date.

A dedicated notebook and pen: The best way to motivate yourself is to record your progress. You are going to write down every aspect of the program until the wedding day, including your meals, exercise challenges, and results. There are detailed instructions in each chapter so you know what to record and when to record it. Use part of the notebook for your daily food diary, in which you will record the calories you have consumed each day. This may sound like a bother, but good results depend upon it.

A scale: Record your body weight before you start this program. Weigh yourself when you are nude, preferably first thing in the morning before you have eaten anything. Record your weight in the journal. Only weigh yourself once a week. Don't drive yourself crazy by checking the scales every day. Your weight naturally fluctuates, and you don't want to psyche yourself out just because you may carrying premenstrual water weight. Remember, the most important way to stay on the plan is by keeping a positive attitude.

NOW THAT I'M NAKED, I SEE CELLULITE!

Cellulite is simply a sign of toxicity and a clogged lymphatic system. Toxins are trapped in the body and present themselves as lumps in the skin, often on the upper thighs and buttocks. The good news is that you can remove cellulite with proper nutrition and loss of excess water. Ironically, the way to get rid of cellulite is to drink plenty of water. By following the one gallon-a-day rule, you can flush the toxins out of your system, and the cellulite will disappear.

A soft cloth tape measure: You'll use this to take your girth measurements. These numbers are useful for evaluating changes in the body. You will need a cloth tape measure. Pressing lightly, measure and record the circumference around the neck, mid biceps (upper arm), mid forearm, the breast at the nipple line, the waist, hips (with feet together), thighs just below the buttocks, and the calf. Try to measure at the same spot every time, using the same arm or leg. Record each of these on a separate line. Then, add all the measurements together to get one total number. Take these measurements every month, and compare both the total number and the individual body parts.

A camera and friendly photographer: Another great motivator is to take a set of full body "before" photographs. Highlight your problem areas by wearing as little clothing as possible. Have someone you love and trust—not the fiancé!—help you take these pictures. Take a front shot, with your arms to the side, a side profile, and a rear view, facing a wall, arms at the side. Glue these photos to your journal, and look at them often. You will take another set of pictures three months before your wedding, and a last set the month before your wedding day. You'll be surprised how quickly your body starts to change.

Food scale and accurate measuring cups: These will allow you to get the portions exact, so you can count your calories. Counting your calories is the key to your weight loss success.

That should do it. Are you tough enough? Not every soldier makes it through boot camp, but you will. By following the program, you should be able to lose one to two pounds per week. So let's get to work!

CHAPTER TWO:
The Hardcore Nutrition Program

While you are preparing for your wedding, the last thing you want to think about is what you eat every day. Yet the foods you consume today affect the way you will look when you walk down the aisle. Body weight is a cumulative process, and your food intake is by far the most important factor determining how you look. It is also the most difficult to control.

The Nutrition Program is a four-part process. The first part determines what your body's energy needs are as defined by the total calories that you consume each day. This number is determined by your age, gender, height, current weight, and metabolism. With this number, you can set a realistic weight loss goal.

The second part is to recognize exactly what you are eating, and how these foods affect your body. You will learn to identify trigger foods, and see why it is important to choose whole, natural foods over processed foods.

The third part is to understand the importance of water. Water not only speeds up waste elimination, but will flush a host of toxins out of your system, as well as aid your diet in countless other ways.

Finally, there are three hardcore meal plans set for intervals of six months, three months, and one month before the wedding. If you have more than fifty pounds to lose, you will need to enter Bootcamp sooner than the six month interval. By following the daily recommendations, you will adopt better eating habits that will lead to immediate weight loss and an overall healthier diet for the future.

PART ONE:
Determine Your Body's Energy Needs

Metabolism is the rate at which all physical and chemical changes take place in the body. The metabolic rate reflects how rapidly the body uses its energy stores, or to put it more bluntly, how quickly you burn calories. Many factors affect this rate, but the most important is your body mass index and your level of exercise.

Basal metabolism or Basal Metabolic Rate (BMR) represents the calories required for fundamental life functions at rest, not including the digestion of food. BMR is the amount of calories you expend by simply lying on your bed, doing nothing.

The Resting Metabolic Rate (RMR) is the BMR plus the additional energy expenditure needed to digest food. RMR is usually 5–10 percent higher than your BMR. If you can estimate your RMR and add your daily activity energy needs, you can determine the estimated daily calories your body needs. This is referred to as the *daily caloric maintenance level*. When you eat at your caloric maintenance level, your body fat will remain stable, and you will neither lose nor gain weight. When you begin to eat below your caloric maintenance level, you will lose body fat.

Once you determine your caloric maintenance level, record it in your journal. You will need to know this number when you begin the hardcore meal plans.

How do you make that determination? I will share two systems. The first, the Harris-Benedict equation, requires a fair amount of math, but it is the most accurate. If you don't want to go through all that trouble, I will suggest a simpler, although less accurate method, below.

The Harris-Benedict equation uses a person's gender, age, weight, and height to arrive at a specific base number. The base number is then multiplied by a second number—ranging from 1.2 for sedentary people to 2.4 for extremely active people—to arrive at the right number of calories. It is very accurate, although a little cumbersome. If you don't want to go through the trouble, I will show you an easier method, below. If you would like to try it, however, here's how to do it:

The Harris-Benedict Equation for Women

Here's the formula:

Basal energy expenditure (B.E.E.) = 655.1 + (9.563 x kg) + (1.850 x cm) – (4.676 x age)

kg = your weight in kilos (your weight divided by 2.2)

cm = your height in centimeters (your height in inches x 2.54)

Note:

1 kg = 2.2 kilos

1 inch = 2.54 centimeters

Example: Carol weighs 160 pounds, is 5'5" and is 30 years old. To find out her B.E.E.

1. First convert her weight into kilos:

160 divided by 2.2. = 73 kilos (rounding off)

2. Next, convert her height into inches:

Given that 12 inches = 1 foot, 5'5" = 65 inches

3. Height in centimeters = height in inches x 2.54

165 centimeters = 65 x 2.54

4. Now to find out Carol's B.E.E.:

B.E.E. = 655.1 + (9.563 x weight in kg) + (1.850 x height in cm) – (4.676 x age)

B.E.E. = 655.1 + (9.563 x 73) + (1.850 x 165) – (4.676 x 30)

B.E.E. = 655.1 + 698 + (305.25) – (140.28)

      =1518

5. Once you determine your basal energy expenditure number, you need to multiply it by the right "activity level multiplier" to determine your calorie maintenance level.

Daily Caloric Maintenance Level = B.E.E. x Activity Level

Activity Level Multiplier

Use:

1.2 if you are sedentary (i.e., little or no exercise, desk job)

1.375 if you are lightly active (i.e., light exercise/sports 1–3 days a week)

1.55 if you are moderately active (i.e., active-moderate exercise/sports 3–5 days/wk)

1.725 if you are extremely active (i.e., hard exercise/sports 6–7 days/wk)

Carol leads a lightly active lifestyle. To find her daily caloric maintenance level, we'd use the following equation:

B.E.E. x 1.375 = Daily caloric maintenance level

1518 x 1.375 = 2087

The Alternative

This system is not as accurate as the Harris-Benedict equation, but it will get you close. It was developed by Edward A. Byrd, current president of the Medical Research Institute. This system uses a simple 14.25 multiplier. In other words:

Your current weight x 14.25 = your daily caloric maintenance level

For example, Carol weighs 160 pounds. 160 x 14.25 = 2280

In order for Carol to maintain her current weight she can consume 2280 calories per day. (Notice that this is a slightly higher number than under the Harris-Benedict formula.) However, think of this number as a moving target: as Carol loses body fat, *her total caloric needs will go down.*

In order to identify how much weight you can potentially lose, you also need to know your body's current makeup: how much of your total weight is fat, and how much is muscle tissue. The goal is to maintain muscle tissue while you lose body fat. If you lose one to two pounds a week, you are primarily loosing body fat. Any more than that and you could begin to lose muscle tissue. For example, if you lose five pounds in one week, you probably lost some water and some lean muscle tissue. You will weigh less, but you will also be flabbier. By measuring your body fat, you keep yourself motivated to stick with the program.

We need a method to determine if the pounds we are losing are muscle or fat. The way we do this is by measuring our body fat percentage. There are many methods used to estimate body fat. By far, the easiest and most popular method is the skinfold caliper technique. The caliper is a hand-held device that determines your skin's density by measuring fat on various parts of the body. When done properly, the results are extremely accurate.

I recommend that you purchase a skinfold caliper. Although many skinfold calipers look similar, each may use a different formula to determine body fat percentage. I recommend the Slim Guide Caliper. It is pretty accurate, and for under twenty-five dollars, it offers the most value for your buck.

Follow the instructions for use carefully. Record your body fat percentage and weight every two weeks in your journal. For the best results, ask someone to help you take the various measurements. Again, not the fiancé! Try to get the same person to perform the tests each time, and try to take the measurements at the exact same location each time.

If you choose not to purchase a skinfold caliper, you can visit your local gym and ask a qualified personal trainer to take your body fat percentage.

Once you know your body fat percentage, you can determine your body composition, which consists of your body fat versus your lean muscle mass. Here is a simple formula to determine your body fat composition:

1. Your current weight x body fat percentage = body fat in pounds
2. Your current weight – body fat in pounds = lean muscle mass in pounds

In our example, Carol weighs 160 pounds, and her body fat is 32 percent.

160 x 32% = 51 pounds of fat

160 – 51 = 108 pounds of lean muscle mass.

Body Fat Percentage Chart for Women

Very lean	under 17%
Fit and lean	18–22%
Average	23–27%
Fair	28–35%
Unhealthy	35%+

Carol has 32 percent body fat, so she falls into the "fair" category. If she wants to lose twenty-five pounds of fat in time for her wedding, she needs to set her sights on lowering her body fat to 20 percent. That would boost her into the "fit and lean" category. Let's say Carol currently weights 160 pounds, as in the example below:

Before:	After:
Weight 160	Weight 135
Body fat 32%	Body fat 20%
Fat 51.2 lb.	Fat 27 lb.
Muscle 108.8 lb.	Muscle 108 lb.

To look your best, you want to keep your muscle tissue intact so you look toned, and not flabby. Realize, however, that if you have a body fat percentage of 35 percent or higher, and you intend to drop a lot of weight before your wedding day, you may not be able to prevent losing some muscle tissue.

That's why it's always better to start a weight loss program early and make the weight loss gradual. Under ideal conditions, you would take the number of calories required to maintain your weight at current levels, and cut it by 20 percent. This would help you trim fat slowly, while only losing a minimal amount of muscle tissue.

But you may not have the time to make your weight loss that gradual. If you have a lot to lose in a short time, you may need to cut calories by 50 percent.

When you are on a weight loss program, it's important to know when you are losing muscle as you are trying to trim down and lose body fat. If you begin to lose muscle you will become flabby, and open the door to eventually gaining the weight back. As you lose weight, check your body fat measurements every two weeks.

For example, in the first three weeks of her diet, Carol lost fifteen pounds. Her body fat was reduced to 30 percent. She was very proud of her accomplishments, until she did the math:

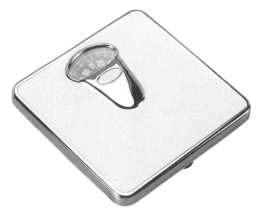

Week	Weight	Body Fat %	Lean Muscle Mass	Body Fat in Pounds
1	160	32	108	51
3	145	30	101	43

Carol lost eight pounds of fat and a whopping seven pounds of lean muscle mass. Even though she was a success on the scale, Carol did not understand that she was doing something wrong. She was either under eating or over exercising, or both. Instead, Carol should have modified her program so that she lost less muscle mass. In other words, she lost too much weight too soon.

Keep yourself motivated by tracking your progress in your journal. Record your body fat every two weeks, your weight every week, and your girth every month. With these numbers in hand, you now have a clear vision for how much weight your body frame can sustain. So, what are you going to eat now?

PART TWO:
What's In Your Mouth?

The key to weight loss is directing the body to use its stored fat as the calories you need for energy. This will reduce existing fat stores. There is really no surprise for how you can achieve this: you need to change what you eat, and how much you are eating.

All foods are comprised of proteins, fats, or carbohydrates. Many foods are a combination of two or more groups. Identifying these groups is a necessary step to weight loss.

Protein

Protein is vital to the growth and development of all body tissues. It is also needed for the formation of hormones, which control a variety of body functions such as growth, sexual development, and metabolic rate. Protein provides 4 calories per gram, and unlike carbohydrates and fats, the body can't store protein. You know the old saying: use it or lose it.

It is generally recommended that protein is 20 to 25 percent of your total caloric intake. If you enjoy eating meats, poultry, and fish, you are probably getting more than enough protein to sustain a healthy diet. If you are a vegetarian, you can create a complete protein meal by combining foods from the grain column with something from either the beans or seeds and nuts columns for two or more meals a day:

Vegetarian Protein Sources

Grain	Beans	Seed and Nuts	Vegetables
Brown rice	Black beans	Split peas	Asparagus
Quinoa	Black-eyed peas	Sunflower seeds	Broccoli
Barley	Chickpeas	Walnuts	Brussels sprouts
Millet	Kidney beans	Cashews	Cabbage
Buckwheat	Soy beans	Nuts	Collard greens
Wheat pasta	Lima beans		Kale
Rice noodles	Lentils		Mustard greens
Breads	Split peas		

The recommended Daily Allowance (RDA) for protein is 0.8 gm/kg/day. Protein requirements increase for physically active adults. If you are physically active you should be consuming 1.2 grams/kg/day per pound of lean body mass. You can determine your lean body mass by doing the following calculations:

Protein Calculations for Physically Active Adults

1. Weight (in pounds) ÷ 2.2 = __ kg
2. Weight in __ kg x 1.2 gm/kg protein= __ gm

Example

Debbie weighs 180 pounds and works out three times a week.

1. 180 lbs ÷ 2.2 = 82 kg
2. 82 x 1.2 = 98 gm protein a day

Debbie should be consuming at least 98 grams of protein. If she eats five times a day, that's 20 grams of protein at each meal.

Carbohydrates

Carbohydrates help regulate the digestion and utilization of protein and fats. Your intake of carbohydrates should be between 50 to 60 percent of your total caloric intake. Like proteins, carbohydrates yield four calories per gram.

Carbohydrates are the chief source of energy for all body functions. Because your body uses so much energy each day, it leads to a rapid depletion of available carbohydrates and creates a continual craving. Those cravings we all have for breads, pasta, pizza, and sweets are not simply in our head. They are actually based on our body's need to create quick energy. This fact alone makes avoiding carbohydrates one of the most difficult parts of weight loss.

Processed carbohydrate snacks contain large amounts of refined sugars and starches. When eaten, they promote a sudden rise in blood sugar levels, providing the body with an immediate source of energy. The rise in blood sugar forces the body to produce an insulin spike, which rapidly lowers the blood sugar levels and results in cravings for more sugary foods. This sugar roller coaster can cause fatigue, dizziness, nervousness, and headaches.

Do yourself a favor: even after the wedding, try to stay away from the following foods:
• White bread
• Bagels
• Donuts
• Soft drinks

- White rice
- Pasta
- Sugar
- Packaged breakfast cereals
- Alcoholic beverages
- Coffee and caffeinated teas

There are plenty of healthy, nutrient-rich carbohydrates to eat that can satisfy your appetite and your body's nutritional requirements. When choosing carbohydrates, complex carbohydrates such as whole grains and vegetable are preferred over simple carbohydrates like the ones mentioned above. Healthy complex carbohydrates include vegetable-based soups, salads, beans, fruits, and whole grains, including barley, bran, hominy, brown rice, whole wheat, bulgur, and rye.

Fiber

Many fruits and whole grains are complex carbohydrates and are excellent sources of fiber. Dietary fiber provides bulk in the diet, which makes you feel full. Fiber-rich foods prevent constipation and establish regular bowel movements. Fiber can also help reduce the risk of colon cancer and diminish risks of heart and artery disease by lowering blood cholesterol. The recommended dietary allowance (RDA) for fiber-rich foods is twenty-five grams a day.

Fats

Fats are the most concentrated source of food energy. One gram of fat yields approximately nine calories, supplying more than twice the calories per gram of carbohydrates or proteins. Fats are essential for the development of cell membranes and hormones and act as a form of insulation. They serve as shock absorbers for our tissues. Dietary fat is essential for that feeling of satiety. Daily fat intake can range from 15 percent to 20 percent.

As with carbohydrates, there are good fats and bad fats. Good fats are found in lean cuts of beef, chicken, fish, lamb, turkey, and dairy products, as well as seeds and flaxseed oil, and omega oils from fish. Bad fats are found in cooking oils, which are used in everything from fried foods to packaged baked goods, including cookies, chips, and store-bought breads. As you can guess, fast food restaurants serve up a basket of unhealthy fat with every meal. Make it a priority to stay away from processed foods in general, and you will automatically cut your fat intake by half.

Controlling Your Cravings

If you want to lose body fat and fit into your dress, you have to control your food cravings. If you have ever tried to lose weight before, you know that you'll start a diet with the best intentions. But pretty soon, you find yourself eating your trigger foods. You know they're forbidden, and they cause you to give up your healthy meal plan for the rest of the day. It comes down to this: the key to successful weight loss is combating your cravings.

We all have problems with certain foods. Many of us use food as a form of self-medication. For example, if you are having a bad day, you might reach for a chocolate bar or a donut. After eating these sweets, your body seems to be calling for a bigger meal to satisfy an empty feeling. The next thing you know, you've made yourself a big steak dinner. After eating a heavy meal, you think a little dessert and coffee will perk you up. Later, you have trouble sleeping so you snack on a bowl of cereal and milk to put you to sleep.

The first step to ending this roller coaster is to understand how food affects our body and mind. There are basically two categories of foods, extreme foods and balanced foods, as noted by Joshua Rosenthal, author of *The Energy Balanced Diet*.

Extreme foods are foods that have an extreme effect on your body, and include sugar and processed foods, as well as red meats and dairy products. All of these extreme foods contribute to the cravings cycle. Eating red meat triggers cravings for sugar and processed foods. Processed foods and sugars lead to cravings for proteins.

By contrast, balanced foods are rich in nutrients. They don't cause craving for more nutrition and are easy to digest. Balanced foods include whole grain products, such as brown rice, quinoa, and tofu, as well as fruits and vegetables.

Don't be hard on yourself for having cravings. Eat extreme foods in moderation. Gradually begin to remove them from your diet, one category at a time.

Satisfying Cravings

If you crave sweets, these natural sweeteners can satisfy any sweet tooth. Pour a small amount on a plain rice cake for a treat that is sweet, crunchy, and low calorie.

- Barley malt
- Honey
- Rice syrup

Read product labels and avoid foods that contain corn syrup, dehydrated cane juice, glucose, dextrose, maltose, or sucrose. These are just different words for table sugar. Instead look for the syrups listed above, or rice syrup.

Cravings for salty food often indicate a craving for minerals. Before you go out and purchase a bag of chips, eat a big green leafy salad. This will often satisfies the craving for salty foods.

In general, your diet should consist of complex carbohydrates in the form of whole grains and vegetables, protein, and healthy fats. This combination will make you feel satisfied, yet keep you away from foods that will surely add on the pounds.

These foods require some preparation. I prepare all of my meals for the week on Sunday and then freeze them. Or, I cook two times during the week. This way my meals are available throughout the day, which prevents me from making poor food choices when I get hungry.

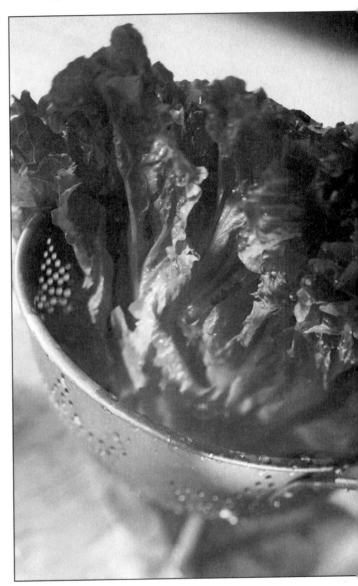

The Bridal Bootcamp™ Four Food Groups

Forget the four food groups you learned about in elementary school. Here in Bridal Bootcamp™ we have our own rules. Create meals that combine food from each group. Consult the various meal plans to show how much of each of these foods you'll be eating before you go shopping: these foods don't have much of a shelf life, and you'll get more out of them when you eat them fresh.

Group 1: Green leafy vegetables: these vegetables are extremely low in calories, and include spinach, asparagus, Brussels sprouts, broccoli, cabbage, mustard greens, and watercress.

Group 2: Sweet vegetables: sweet potatoes, parsnips, pumpkins, squash, carrots, and white fleshed potatoes.

Group 3: Proteins: meat, chicken, fish, eggs, and soy products.

Group 4: Whole grains: brown rice, barley, buckwheat, corn, millet, and wheat berries.

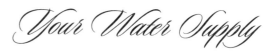

PART THREE:
Your Water Supply

Is all this good eating making you thirsty? Reach for a glass of water, or maybe more. You should drink three quarts of water per day. Water intake should also be increased when you are exercising or if you live in a hot climate.

Drinking water helps your body metabolize stored fat: it acts as a stimulus in decreasing fat deposits and keeps the excess off. Water also helps rid the body of metabolic toxins and waste, which will improve your energy levels.

Drinking lots of water is probably the best thing you can do for your body. Here are a few more reasons why:

- Water improves endocrine gland function
- By drinking lots of water, fluid retention is alleviated (funny how that happens)
- Liver function improves, therefore increasing the percentage of fat used for energy
- Natural thirst returns
- Metabolic functions improve
- Water helps eliminate waste and detoxifies pollutants from your body

- Water keeps skin flawless.
- Water helps muscles maintain the ability to contract and keep good tone
- Appetite decreases significantly

I recommend that you drink pure spring water or distilled water throughout the day. In the morning, drink eight ounces of warm—more than room temperature—water mixed with the juice of one lemon, followed by another eight ounces of room temperature water. This will help clean out your liver and eliminate waste. Nothing helps you shed pounds like extra waste elimination.

Start with four 8-ounce glasses per day. After one week, move up to eight 8-ounce glasses daily. The next week, shoot for one gallon per day. Start drinking your water in the morning before breakfast, and then continue drinking throughout the day. Also, drink plenty of water before, during, and after exercise, and whenever you feel hungry. However, do not drink water with your meals. This will slow digestion. Instead, drink either thirty minutes before meals, or wait thirty minutes after eating to drink.

PART FOUR:
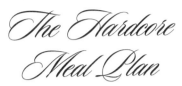
The Hardcore Meal Plan

You've gone shopping. Your refrigerator and pantry are full. You've set goals for pounds to be shed. You have a glass of water handy. Now you're ready for the hardcore meal plans.

These meal plans are based on a calorie-counting program featuring nutritious and satisfying meals. The six, three, and one month workouts each contain their own special meal plans.

You will be eating five meals each day. We have provided seven-day meal plans for your convenience. You may use them, or use the meals provided as a guide to show you how to mix the appropriate four groups to get to the proper rations of 50 percent carbohydrates, 30 percent protein, 20 percent fat. Use a calorie counting book like Corrine T. Netzer's, *The Complete Book of Food Counts*, so that you can make the exchanges. This is a great book which contains the nutritional breakdown of many raw and processed foods.

The meal plans are all broken down as follows:

Meal 1 Breakfast

Meal 2 Mid-morning snack

Meal 3 Lunch

Meal 4 Afternoon snack

Meal 5 Dinner

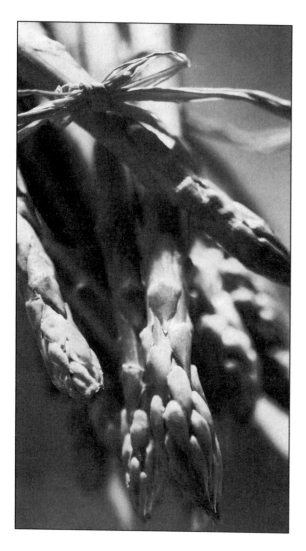

Hardcore Rules of the Road

No matter when you begin, there are several rules that apply:

- Divide your total calorie allotment into five small meals each day, eating every three hours. Eating small, frequent meals will not only speed up your metabolism, they provide the key to preserving muscle. This pattern of eating will also keep blood sugar levels stable, and keep you from feeling hungry.

- Your diet should consist of approximately 50 percent carbohydrate, 30 percent protein, 20 percent fat every meal. This balance will help to maintain stable blood sugar levels, and fuel muscles with nutrients.

- Do not skip meals. That hungry feeling eventually leads to poor food choices later in the day.

- Consume the proper amount of calories. Do not under-eat significantly below your allotted calorie count.

- Carry a bottle of water with you wherever you go, and drink frequently throughout the day.

- Be certain to have food from your meal plan available at work, home, school and when traveling.

- Don't worry about eating late at night, as long as you are eating the required amount of calories per day.

- Cut down on alcohol. There are 150 calories in a bottle of beer or one glass of wine!

- Learn to read food labels. Remember we are counting calories, not carbohydrates. Fat and/ or carbohydrates do not make you gain weight; excess calories do.

- Stay away from trigger foods and extreme foods, especially processed foods.

- Make a grocery list before you go food shopping. And never shop when you're hungry: you'll end up buying all the wrong kinds of foods.

- Keep a food diary in your journal. Write down tomorrow's meals the night before and the times you plan to eat them. Write down what you ate immediately after each meal, and tally up your total calories at the end of the day.

- If you go over your daily allotment, cut back on calories toward the end of the day. But don't skip a meal!

- If you binge during the week write down precisely what you did and how you felt just before you ate. It should become obvious what triggers that behavior. If you are stressed and feel compelled to binge, try to do something, at that very moment, that will distract you. Take a walk, talk to a friend, go exercise. Walk away from the refrigerator!

- Do not weigh yourself without measuring your body fat. The scale may not have budged, but your body fat percent may have decreased, which means your muscle weight has increased.

- Chew your food consciously, fifteen to twenty times per bite. It will aid in digestion.

- If you get hungry late at night, drink more water: it will fill you up. Don't worry about going to the bathroom in the middle of the night. The more water you drink, the more efficiently your body eliminates waste. The first few nights might be a problem, but it is still better than eating extra calories.

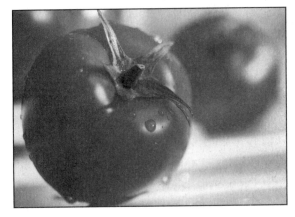

I DON'T HAVE TIME FOR THIS!
THE ULTIMATE MEAL REPLACEMENT GUIDE

If you don't have time to prepare healthy and nutritious meals, meal replacement bars and shakes are not a bad solution. They're a quick and convenient way to get a lot of high quality protein, carbohydrates, and a host of other important nutrients. Use them for meals 2 and 4 as a variety of snack.

There are many meal replacement bars and shakes on the market. But whole foods are always better than anything in powder form. Though you can buy meal replacements at your local health food store, you can also easily make your own. Follow the directions for one of my smoothie and protein recipes listed on the following pages.

The most important ingredient in any homemade meal replacement is protein. Of all the proteins out there, whey protein is no doubt the best. Whey proteins are high quality proteins that come from milk. Whey protein contains many similar ingredients to those found in breast milk. It supplies the body with many essential amino acids needed for good health. Whey proteins are used by athletes to repair and build muscles after a tough workout. There are two I recommend. One is Iso-Pure Zero Carbs, a whey protein supplement. It has 100 calories per scoop and 25 grams of protein. The other is Gotein, which is a good source of protein. It has 55 calories per scoop and 120 grams of protein.Made from pure goat milk, this is a good substitute for people who cannot digest cow's milk. It also contains all the essential amino acids and is minimally processed to preserve its original composition.

On those occasions when you don't have time to make your own protein snack, beware of protein bars. Back in 2001, Consumer labs studied the contents of these bars and determined that eighteen of the thirty bars tested failed to meet their labeling claims. On average, these bars exceeded their sugar claims by 8 grams, which is equivalent to two teaspoons. So when you shop for protein bars, always read the labels. Some will contain glycerin, an ingredient that is not counted in the total carbohydrate content. When you are shopping for protein bars, choose ones that have whole food ingredients: try the selection at your local health food store instead of the supermarket.

Homemade, Whole Food, Protein Shakes and Smoothies

The following recipes use all natural ingredients to create delicious snacks. Add whey protein or goat protein so that you can meet your protein requirements for that meal. My favorite is Gotein: Pure Goat's Milk Protein by Garden of Life. Also consider using vanilla-flavored soy milk or rice milk, instead of cow's milk. Cow milk molecules are large and hard to digest for most people. Even though milk is loaded with calcium, you won't get any of the benefits if you are among those people who can't digest cow's milk.

If you are still want to use cow's milk, try to find organic milk, which is free from chemicals, antibiotics, or hormones, yet contains all of the same vitamins.

The Recipes

Peanut Butter Paradise

8 ounces organic fat-free milk, or organic soy milk

1 banana

$^1/_2$ tablespoon peanut butter

1 scoop Gotein protein supplement ($^1/_2$ scoop if you are using Iso-Pure)

2 ice cubes

Calories 369

Protein 22.42

Carbohydrates 48.3

Fat 9.55

Place all the ingredients in a blender in the order listed. Blend on a high speed for one minute. The consistency should be smooth like a milk shake.

Tip: To increase your fiber intake, you can add a $^1/_4$ cup of wheat bran to each Smoothie recipe. This will add 30 calories to the recipe.

Berry Blend Smoothie

12 ounces organic low fat milk, or organic soy milk

½ cup blueberries

½ cup raspberries

½ tablespoon honey

1 scoop Gotein protein supplement (½ scoop if you are using Iso-Pure)

2 ice cubes

Calories 386

Protein 23.58

Carbohydrates 54.95

Fat 8.12

Place all the ingredients into a blender in the order listed. If fresh fruit is not in season, substitute with unsweetened frozen fruit. And reduce the ice requirement to one ice cube. Blend on a high speed for one minute. The consistency should be icy like a smoothie.

Strawberry Fields

8 ounces apple juice

2 ounces water

1 cup strawberries

½ banana

¼ cup low fat vanilla yogurt

2 tsp flaxseed oil

1 scoop Gotein protein supplement (½ scoop if you are using Iso-Pure)

2 ice cubes

Calories 434

Protein 19.64

Carbohydrates 63.14

Fat 12.17

Place all the ingredients into a blender in the order listed. If fresh strawberries are not in season, substitute with unsweetened frozen strawberries. And reduce the ice requirement to one ice cube. Blend on a high speed for one minute. The consistency should be icy like a smoothie.

The Cleanser

6 ounces cranberry juice

3 ounces water

1/2 banana

1/2 cup fresh blueberries

1/2 cup fresh strawberries

1 tablespoon honey

2 scoops Gotein protein supplement (1 scoop if you are using Iso-Pure)

2 ice cubes

Calories 379

Protein 28.21

Carbohydrates 54.73

Fat 6.38

Place all the ingredients into a blender in the order listed. If fresh fruits are not in season, substitute unsweetened frozen fruit. And reduce the ice requirement to one ice cube. Blend on a high speed for one minute. The consistency should be icy like a smoothie.

Brazilian Rain

4 ounces unsweetened pineapple juice

4 ounces unsweetened orange juice

2 ounces water

1/2 cup fresh mango chunks

2 scoops Gotein supplement (1 scoop if you are using Iso-Pure)

2 ice cubes

Calories 390

Protein 25.8

Carbohydrates 51.8

Fat 9.71

Place all the ingredients into a blender in the order listed. If fresh mango is not in season, substitute unsweetened frozen mango. And reduce the ice requirement to one ice cube. Blend on a high speed for one minute. The consistency should be icy like a smoothie.

Java Junkies

12 ounces organic fat-free milk, or organic soy milk

$1/2$ banana

1 tablespoon peanut butter

1 tablespoon instant coffee

1 scoop Gotein protein ($1/2$ scoop if you are using Iso-Pure)

2 ice cubes

Calories 422

Protein 24.15

Carbohydrates 53.8

Fat 13.27

Place all the ingredients into a blender in the order listed. Blend on a high speed for one minute. The consistency should be smooth like a milk shake.

The American

12 ounces organic fat-free milk

3 tablespoons rolled oats or oatmeal

1 tablespoon almond butter or peanut butter

1 banana

1 scoop Gotein protein supplement ($1/2$ scoop if you are using Iso-Pure)

2 ice cubes

Calories 444

Protein 32.67

Carbohydrates 58.7

Fat 10.21

Place all of the ingredients into a blender in the order listed. Blend on a high speed for one minute. The consistency should be smooth like a milk shake.

Dessert Surprise: Strawberry Granola Fruit Parfait

6 ounces low fat vanilla yogurt

5 strawberries, sliced

¼ cup blueberries

½ cup granola

Calories 359

Protein 17.33

Carbohydrates 53.53

Fat 9.94

In an 8-ounce cup, layer one tablespoon of granola at the bottom, then add half of the nonfat vanilla yogurt, and place in a few slices of strawberries. Add another layer of granola, yogurt, and more strawberries. Repeat until all of the ingredients are used in two tiers. Sprinkle the remaining granola on top and garnish with a strawberry slice.

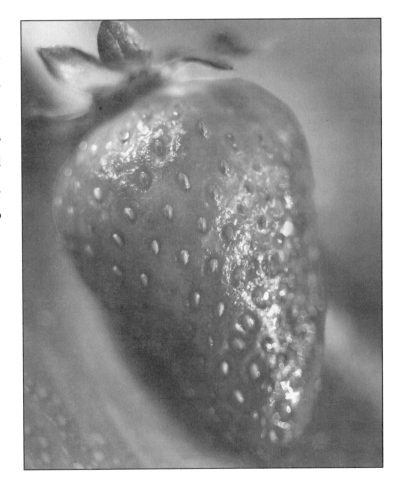

CHAPTER THREE:

The Bridal Bootcamp™ Supplement Program

The typical American diet falls short of the RDA for nutrients. Once you forego junk foods and processed foods and switch to a balanced diet based on natural, whole foods, you can still destroy the nutrients during the cooking process. What's a girl to do?

As you countdown to the wedding, watching your calories, a multivitamin/mineral complex supplement will make sure that you get the nutrients you need.

All women need to take a broad-spectrum, balanced multivitamin/multimineral supplement, which contains all of the essential vitamins and trace minerals. In most cases, you will need to supplement this multivitamin with additional calcium and magnesium.

While there are many vitamin manufacturers, there are basically four types of multivitamin supplements to choose from. The difference between them is how many times a day they should be taken and whether or not they contain adequate levels of calcium and magnesium.

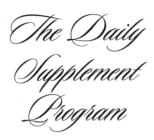

The Daily Supplement Program

One per day multivitamin: While a single pill seems quick and convenient, this type of product has one major disadvantage: most of the nutrients in a single dose multivitamin are water soluble. This means that any excess vitamin that cannot be processed immediately will be eliminated. Most of the content is absorbed in an hour or two and metabolized and excreted in two or three more hours. This means that if you take your vitamins with breakfast, by lunchtime, most of the nutrients you took will be gone. Also, the amount of calcium and magnesium required is too large to fit into one tablet.

Two per day multivitamin: For multivitamins, two is always better than the one, assuming that one tablet is taken in the morning and the other in the evening. But, this type of product still does not contain enough calcium and magnesium.

Complete (four to six per day) multivitamin and multimineral: These are the way to go if you do not want to compromise your supplement intake but you want the convenience of taking one product. With a recommended daily dose of four tablets or six capsules, you will also ingest meaningful amounts of calcium and magnesium.

Specialty Multivitamins and Herbal Supplements: From a marketing standpoint, this category is very popular. There are high energy formulas and a variety of age specific women's formulas. But you have to be careful not to lose sight of what is really important— the essential vitamins and minerals. In other words, remember that your multivitamin should contain adequate amounts of all the essential vitamins and minerals. And if you want a secondary product containing additional nutrients, that's fine. Just be careful that these extra ingredients do not take the place of the essential nutrients in your daily supplement.

I recommend the two per day multivitamin approach, combined with a separate calcium/magnesium supplement also taken twice per day. Your two per day tablets should contain the following vitamins and trace minerals at minimum:

Beta-carotene (vitamin A)	25,000 International Unit (IU)
Vitamin D (from natural form vitamin D3)	400 IU
Vitamin C	500 milligram (mg)
Natural Vitamin E (succinate)	400 mg
Vitamin B1 (thiamine)	25 mg
Vitamin B2 (riboflavin)	25 mg
Vitamin B6 (pyridoxine)	25 mg
Vitamin B12 (cobalamin)	100 mg
Niacinamide	100 mg
Pantothenic Acid	50 mg
Biotin	300 microgram (mcg)
Folic Acid	400 mcg
PABA (para-aminobenzoic acid)	25 mg
Choline Bitartrate	25 mg
Inositol	25 mg
Calcium (from calcium citrate and calcium carbonate)	25 mg
Magnesium (from magnesium aspartate and magnesium oxide)	7.2 mg
Potassium (potassium aspartate and Potassium citrate)	5 mg
Zinc (from zinc picolinate)	30 mg
Copper (from copper gluconate)	2 mg
Iron (from ferrous fumarate)	10 mg
Manganese (from manganese gluconate)	5 mg
Iodine (from potassium iodide)	150 mcg
Selenium (from selenomethionine and Selenate (50/50 mixture)	200 mcg
Chromium (GTF)	200 mcg
Molybdenum (from natural molybdic acid)	150 mcg

Calcium and Magnesium

The next most important components of your supplement program are calcium and magnesium. Calcium is an essential mineral. We all know that it plays an important role in maintaining our bones and teeth, but for women, calcium supplements are the number one way to prevent osteoporosis. For women under age 35, calcium is needed to build bone density. After 35, your bone density starts to decline, and calcium is again needed to slow down the process. So, if you are going to do one good thing now for your senior years, start taking these supplements. Be sure that you purchase a calcium supplement that also contains magnesium. You need the magnesium so that your body can absorb the calcium. You need to take at least 1000 milligrams of calcium/magnesium per day, split up in two dosages. Buy calcium/mag supplements in 500 milligrams tablets.

Antioxidants

Now that we have satisfied the foundation requirements and added calcium and magnesium, we can begin customizing your program to meet a bride's unique needs. As an active woman on a weight loss program, you need to take an additional product: an antioxidant blend.

Antioxidants are substances that neutralize unstable molecules in your body that can cause damage. These molecules are sometimes referred to as free radicals, and become unstable because they have an unbalanced internal structure. This unbalance can lead them to attack other molecules causing havoc in your body. Antioxidants are substances that function to block these dangerous free radicals. Cancer, arthritis, atherosclerosis, cataracts, and Parkinson's Disease are all conditions that may result from the damage caused by free radicals.

In addition to the well known antioxidants (vitamin C, vitamin E, beta-carotene, and selenium), there are phytochemicals such as flavonoids, including lycopene, letuin, quercetin, catechins, polyphenols, anthocyanins. These flavonoids are now being recognized as perhaps even more powerful antioxidants than vitamins C and E.

Antioxidants work best when they are used in combination. One of the most basic antioxidant combination formulas is the "ACE" group, because it contains the three basic antioxidant vitamins: A, C, and E. When choosing an antioxidant, look for a product that contains the following minimum allotments:

Vitamin A (as 100% natural beta-carotene from D. salina)	11,000 IU
Vitamin C (as l-ascorbic acid)	600 mg
Vitamin E (d-alpha tocopheryl succinate)	250 IU
Zinc (as zinc aspartate)	22 mg
Selenium (as L-selenomethionine)	75 mcg
L-Cysteine (as L-cysteine HCl)	100 mg
L-Glutathione	25 mg
Carotenoid mix (alpha-carotene, lutein, zeaxanthin, cryptoxanthin)	125 mcg

Taking Vitamins

The best way to take any type of supplements is with food. This prevents ulcers, and leads to the total absorption of the vitamins. I suggest that you take the supplements throughout the day during your meals, as follows:

Morning meal 1: 1 tablet multivitamin

1 tablet calcium/mag

Afternoon meal 3: 1 tablet multivitamin

1 tablet calcium/mag

Evening meal 5: 1 tablet antioxidant

Now you know the drill. If you want to lose fat, you must expend more calories than you consume. The Bridal Bootcamp™ Supplement Program will insure that you receive all the sufficient nutrients to maintain good health. If you don't eat properly and get the nutrients you need, you will be tempted to binge. And if you do binge, you won't see results and will lose your motivation to continue.

Stop the vicious cycle! Get on the right track. Get your diet and supplement program going for one full week. See how great you'll feel. Then, begin the challenges of the wedding workouts.

CHAPTER FOUR:

Fitness Maneuvers: Learning the Exercises

Are you ready to get fit? Now that you know what—and how—to eat during Bridal Bootcamp™, it's time to acquaint yourself with the exercises. The Bridal Bootcamp™ Fitness Program draws from more than eighty different exercises. Each day uses different combinations from the five basic exercise groups: warm-ups, abdominal exercises, strength training, cardiovascular, and cool-down stretches.

Each workout is designed to last an hour. Although the workouts vary, they all follow a standard pattern:

- 10 minute warm-up and dynamic stretching
- 5 minute abdominal drills
- 20 minute strength training
- 20 minute cardiovascular interval session
- 5 minute post-workout stretching

If you start six months before your wedding, you will follow one program for three months. Then, the difficulty and frequency of the workouts will increase as you get closer to the wedding. The month before the wedding is the most intense, ending with a period of total rest the week before the wedding.

In this chapter, you will find instructions for all of the exercises I use in each of the programs. (You will find the workout programs on page 189, 223, and 255.) Take some time to familiarize yourself with these. No doubt, you will refer back to this section off when you are first learning the exercises.

Why There Are So Many Exercises

Because I am the director of fitness at a Gold's Gym, I designed the program using the resources available to me—namely, standard exercise machines you will find in any well-equipped gym. But don't worry if you don't belong to a gym. I have included exercises you can substitute so you get the full workout at home. The at-home exercises are clearly labeled.

One reason I have included so many exercises in this chapter is to give you that option. Another is to give you an absolutely comprehensive program that will work every muscle. The third reason is that the variety will keep you from getting bored. If you stay interested, you are more likely to continue.

These workouts will make you feel great. After a short time, you will feel like you can conquer the world, not just the reception line. They will also help you lose body fat and increase lean muscle mass.

A Proper Warm-Up

A proper warm-up is essential for a safe and productive workout. Ultimately, you want to bring your heart rate up to 60 percent of your maximum heart rate. You will always start with five minutes of light cardiovascular exercises, followed by full body stretching. (I will explain your cardiovascular exercise options later, when I outline the specific workouts.)

Then you will proceed to a specific set of stretching exercises, drawn from the group that follows. Be sure to note the part of the body for which the stretch is intended. This way you can make sure you feel the stretch specifically in that area.

Here are some tips to help you stretch safely and effectively:

- Warm up. Before you stretch, your muscles should be warm.

- Do not bounce. Bouncing stresses joints, ligaments, and muscles. It also triggers the protective stretch mechanism within each muscle to reflexively contract. As a result, the muscles cannot relax or stretch. Always stretch slowly and gently.

- Breathe. Deep abdominal breathing helps to improve circulation to muscle tissues. It also helps you relax. Holding your breath will make any stretch ineffective.

- Stretch both sides. If you notice that a muscle on one side is tighter than the same muscle on the other side, you should stretch it twice as much to fully relax it. This will create balance and symmetry.

The Warm-Up Exercises

WARM-UPS FOR THE SIX-MONTH WORKOUT

Flutter Kick

Benefits:

This exercise will work your abdominals and warm-up your legs.

To start:

Lie on your back. Place your hands behind your lower back for support. Elevate your head and feet 5 inches from the floor. Keep your head aligned with your body, so you do not strain your neck muscles.

Instructions:

1. Kick your feet up and down as if you were swimming.

2. Continue for 30 seconds.

Mountain Climbers

Benefits:

This exercise will stretch and warm up your thighs and buttocks.

To start:

Get in a push-up position, with your hands directly under your shoulders. Draw your navel inward, with your head facing the floor. Align your head with your spine.

Instructions:

1. Bring your left knee in toward your chest.

2. Then kick the left leg back while simultaneously bringing the right knee toward your chest.

3. Continue this motion for 30 seconds.

Walking Lunge with Twist

Benefits:

This exercise will warm up and stretch your thighs and torso.

To start:

Stand with your feet shoulder width apart, and your arms extended to your sides. Draw your navel inward.

Instructions:

1. Step forward descending slowly to the floor so that your knees form a 90-degree angle.

2. Slowly raise your arms and hands to touch and rotate at the spine to the forward leg side.

3. Use your hip and thigh muscles to push back up to the next step.

4. Rotate the spine back to the starting position.

5. Repeat on the other side.

6. Walk the length of a room twice.

Squat Thrusts

Benefits:

This exercise will warm up your thighs and buttocks.

To start:

Stand with your feet shoulder width apart, toes pointing straight ahead. Draw your navel inward.

Instructions:

1. Flex your knees and hips to slowly lower your body as if you were sitting in a chair. Your knees should not go past your toes, your buttocks should move back and down, and your torso should incline forward 45 degrees.

2. As you come back up to the starting point rotate you hips forward and squeeze your glutes, the large muscles of the buttocks.

3. Continue this exercise for 30 seconds.

Jumping Jacks

Benefits:

This exercise will stretch and warm up your entire body.

To start:

Stand erect with your feet together. Draw your navel inward. Keep your arms at your sides.

Instructions:

1. Jump your feet apart, and at the same time bring your hands together over head.

2. Jump back to the starting position.

3. Continue for 2 minutes.

WARM-UPS FOR THE THREE-MONTHS WORKOUT

Prisoner Squats

Benefits: This exercise will warm up and stretch your thighs and buttocks.

To start: Stand tall with proper alignment, placing your hands behind your head. Keep your navel drawn inward.

Instructions:

1. Lower to a squat position slowly and under control, as you extend your hips, knees and ankles.

2. Rise to a standing position.

3. Do 3 sets, 15 repetitions.

Single-Leg Squat Touchdown

Benefits: This exercise will stretch your lower back, hamstrings, and buttocks.

To start: Stand upright, arms at your sides, draw your navel inward, balancing on one leg.

Instructions:

1. Bend at the hip and touch your toe with your opposite hand. Do not let standing knee move.

2. Slowly return to the starting position.

3. Do 3 sets, 15 repetitions.

Arm Circles

Benefits: This exercise will warm up your shoulders.

To start: Start in a standing position with hands held straight out to your sides. Draw your navel in.

Instructions:

1. Begin moving your arms forward in circles, starting with small ones and getting larger as you progress.

2. Continue for 40 seconds. Stop and repeat by circling in the opposite direction.

Yoga Stretches: Plank Posture with Downward Facing Dog

Benefits:

These yoga postures stretch out your shoulders, chest, and thighs.

To start:

Sit on the floor resting on your hands and knees.

Instructions:

1. Form a table top with your back. Make sure your knees are aligned directly under your hips and your hands are aligned directly under your shoulders.

2. Straighten your legs back behind you, one at a time, forming one line from your head to your toes, resting totally on your hands and feet with arms fully extended. This is the Plank Posture.

3. Come up on your toes and slowly begin straightening your legs to push your hips upward; as your legs straighten, drop your head down toward the ground. Keep your arms straight and elbows relaxed.

4. Try to lower your heels to the floor as your legs straighten; your feet should be about 1 foot apart. Without straining or locking your elbows or knees, create a 90-degree angle with your body, as you make a straight line from your heels to your hips and another from your hips down your arms and to your hands. This posture is called Downward Facing Dog.

5. Do 10 repetitions of 6 full cycles.

Medicine Ball Rotations

Benefits:

These rotations stretch your torso.

To start:

From a standing position, place feet hip-width apart, knees slightly bent and feet straight ahead. Draw your navel in.

Instructions:

1. Hold a medicine ball with both hands and keep elbows fully extended.

2. Initiate the rotational movement from the trunk, moving side to side.

3. Allow the hips to pivot on the back foot as the motions nears end-range.

Note: If your gym does not have a medicine ball, use a five-pound weighted plate, held firmly.

WARM-UPS FOR THE ONE-MONTH WORKOUT

Starburst

Benefits:

This exercise will warm up and stretch your entire body.

To start:

Stand with your feet together, with your arms next to your sides.

Instructions:

1. Jump up and spread your legs in the air, while simultaneously extending your arms out to your sides to about chest height. Land with your feet together, and arms back alongside your body.

2. Perform 10 repetitions.

Kick-Out with Jumping Jacks

Benefits:

This exercise will warm up and stretch your entire body.

To start:

Stand with your feet together, with your arms alongside your body.

Instructions:

1. Drop to the floor placing your hands directly under your shoulders.

2. Kick your legs out behind you, forming a plank with your body.

3. Quickly bring your legs back to start and stand up.

4. Jump and spread your legs open while simultaneously extending your arms over your ears, bringing your hands together.

5. Perform 10 repetitions.

Hip Swing

Benefits: This exercise will stretch your thighs, hips, and buttocks.

To start: Stand alongside a wall. Place one hand on the wall.

Instructions:

1. Draw your navel inward.

2. Swing your right leg forward, with control, while your left arm touches your right leg.

3. Swing leg backward. Keep your midsection tight.

4. Repeat on the opposite leg.

5. Do 10 repetitions on each leg.

Jumping Squats

Benefits:

This exercise strengthens and shapes your entire legs and buttocks.

To start:

Stand with your legs slightly wider than shoulder width apart. Your torso should be erect with your arms crossed in front of you.

Instructions:

1. Bend your knees and lower into a squat so that your thighs are parallel to the floor. Do not allow your knees to go over your toes.

2. Then jump straight into the air. Land with your feet firmly on the floor descending into another squat.

3. Do 10 repetitions.

Note: This is not a warm up exercise. You will use this during specific strength-training routines.

The Abdominal Exercises

Heart Rate: 55 % of maximum heart rate

The muscle group most commonly referred to as the abdominals allows you to bend at your waist, twist, and keep your torso stable. The abdominal muscles are interconnected to the movement of virtually the entire body so it's very important to build a strong midsection.

A good abdominal routine varies in order to work all of the muscles. It is not possible to isolate the upper abdominal region from the lower. However, you can emphasize one area over the other with certain exercises. By keeping your upper torso stable and raising your legs, you are targeting your lower abdominal region. And if you curve your upper body toward your lower body, the upper abdominals work more strongly. The third section of your routine should work your obliques, the muscles you use when you rotate or bend your body to the opposite side.

Here are some tips to help you do the exercises safely and make the most of them:

- Because the actual range of motion in many abdominal exercises is fairly small, these crunches will be most effective if you use a controlled pace and flex your abdominals hard at the top of each crunch.
- Don't come all the way down to the floor at the bottom of the movement. That would allow you to rest unintentionally between repetitions.
- You will need an exercise or yoga mat.
- Perform the different abdominal routines on each of your training days.
- Perform the exercises together as a set, rest for 20 seconds before performing the next set of exercises. To make the exercises more difficult and stimulate muscle growth, add resistance to your abdominal routine.

THE ABDOMINAL WARM-UP

Before performing any abdominal routine you need to stretch your abdominals. Lay over a physioball and stretch your upper body as far back as possible, maximizing the stretch in your abdominals without causing injury. If your gym does not have a ball, do a yoga Cobra Posture.

Yoga Cobra Posture

To start:

Lie down on your stomach, arms by your sides, palms-up. Turn your head forward, resting your chin on the floor. Bend your elbows, placing your hands up under your shoulders. Your feet are pointed, yet relaxed.

Instructions:

1. On an inhalation, start slowly raising your shoulders and torso off the floor.

2. Lift up as high as is comfortable. Keep your toes pointed and strive to leave your hips on the floor, feet together.

3. When you reach your maximum comfortable stretch hold for 20 seconds. Then lower your torso back to the floor.

ABDOMINAL EXERCISES YOU CAN DO AT HOME

Cross Body Crunch, 58

Basic Crunch, 59

Oblique Crunch, 60

Double Crunch, 61

Cross Over Split-Leg Crunch, 62

Butterfly Crunch, 63

Thigh-Slide Crunch, 64

V-Ups, 65

Scissors Kick, 66

Side Bend, 67

Reverse Crunch with Physioball, 68

Bent Leg Hip-Raise, 69

Bicycle, 70

Hands Over Head Crunch, 71

Figure Four Crunch, 72

Twisting Crunch on the Physioball, 73

Hip Thrust, 74

Reverse Crunch, 75

Side Jackknife, 76

Cross Body-Crunch

To start:

Lie on your back, with your right foot crossed over the left knee, left foot on the floor. Place your hand loosely behind your head.

Instructions:

1. Raise your left shoulder blade off the floor heading across your body toward the outside of your right knee. Go only as far as your body will allow, without straining your neck.

2. Contract your obliques as you go through the movement. Lower your torso back to the starting position.

3. Repeat for the required number of repetitions, then change your legs, and do the other side.

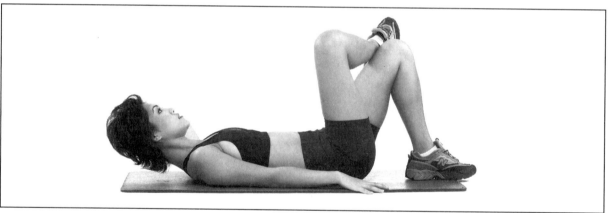

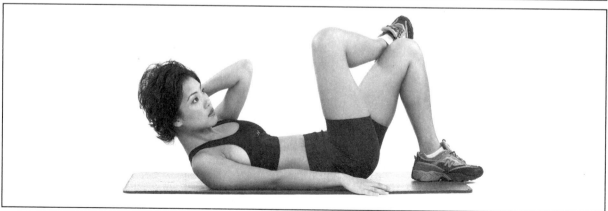

Basic Crunch

To start:

Lie with your back pressing against the floor. Place your hands loosely behind your head, knees bent, feet flat on the floor. Do not pull on your neck. Look up to the ceiling. Imagine that you have placed a tennis ball underneath your chin.

Instructions:

1. Begin to curl your upper body 2 inches off the floor.

2. Contract your abdominal muscles on the way up by bringing your ribcage toward your pelvis. Do not let your shoulder blades touch the floor.

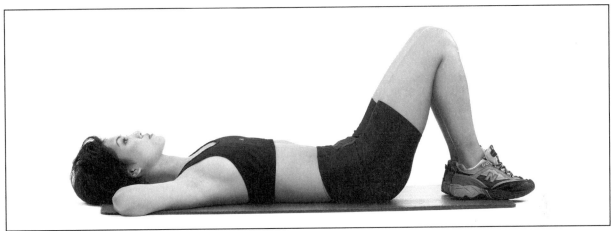

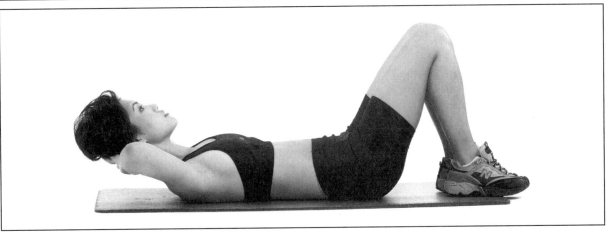

Oblique Crunch

To start:

Lie on the floor on your right side, with your knees bent and legs on top of each other. Place your left hand on your head. Lean on your right arm.

Instructions:

1. Begin to bend your body toward your legs, crunching your obliques as you move.

2. Repeat the required number of repetitions, then change and continue on the other side.

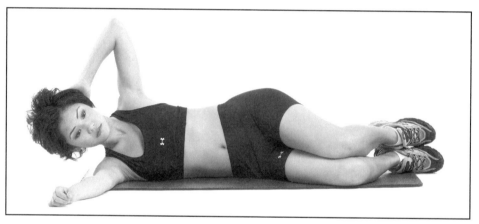

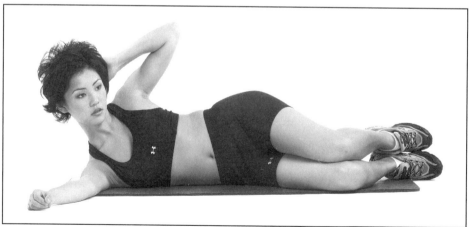

Double Crunch

To start:

Lie on your back with your hands loosely behind your head. Lift your legs off the floor so that your knees form a 90-degree angle.

Instructions:

1. Curl your shoulder blades off the floor while simultaneously bringing your knees toward and over your chest.

2. Contract your abdominals hard.

3. Slowly lower back to the starting position.

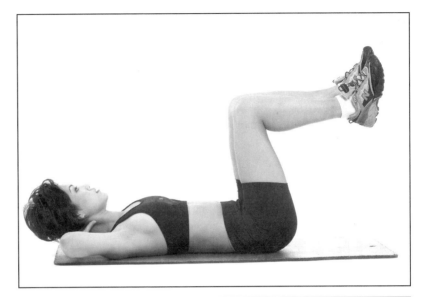

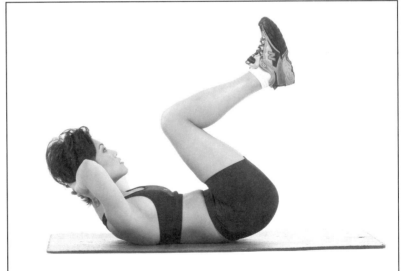

Cross Over Split-Leg Crunch

To start:

Lie down on the floor, legs up in the air and opened a little more than shoulder width apart. Place your arms alongside your body.

Instructions:

1. Curl your upper body and rotate your left arm and shoulder toward to the opposite foot.
2. Lower to the starting position. Repeat on the other side.

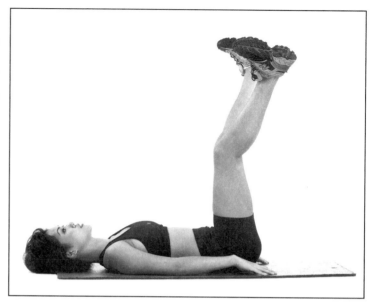

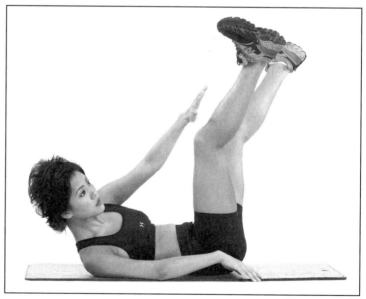

Butterfly Crunch

To start:

Lie on your back, with your knees out to your sides. Your knees should be as close to the floor as possible, with heels touching on the floor. Your hands should be behind your head. Place your hands loosely behind your head.

Instructions:

1. Begin to curl your upper body two inches off the floor.
2. Contract your abdominal muscles on the way up by bringing your ribcage toward your pelvis. Do not let your shoulder blades touch the floor.

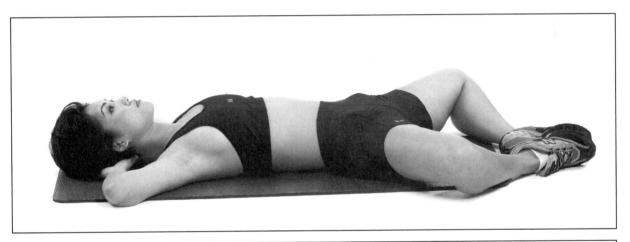

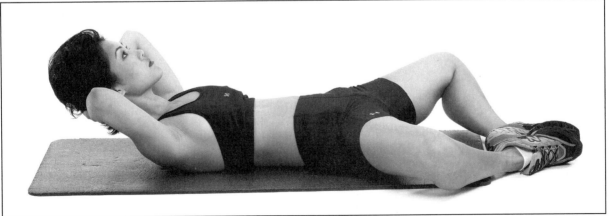

Thigh-Slide Crunch

To start:

Lie on your back with your hands on top of your thighs, legs bent 60 degrees and feet flat on the floor.

Instructions:

1. Curl your head forward and raise your shoulders off the floor, sliding your arms down your thighs.

2. Squeeze your abdominal muscles at the top of the movement.

3. Slowly lower back to the starting position.

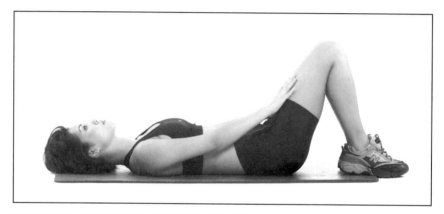

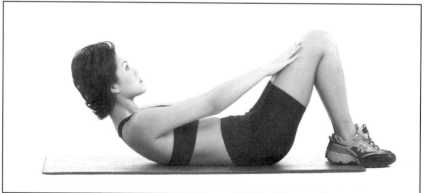

V-Ups

To start:

Lie on the floor with your arms straight at your sides. Raise your upper body off the floor while also lifting your legs up to the same height. Balance on your buttocks.

Instructions:

1. Draw your upper body and your knees toward each other with your arms out in front of you.

2. Squeeze your abdominals and then lengthen your body completely.

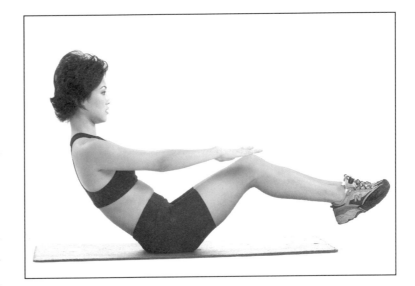

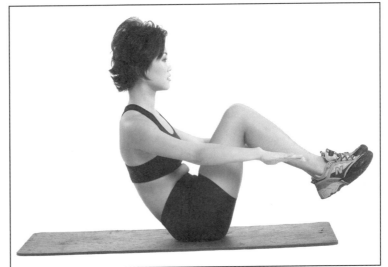

Scissors Kick

To start:

Lie on your back with your arms outstretched at your sides.

Instructions:

1. Lift your legs off the floor and point your toes. Bend your knees slightly.

2. Open your legs and cross them over each other at a fairly slow pace.

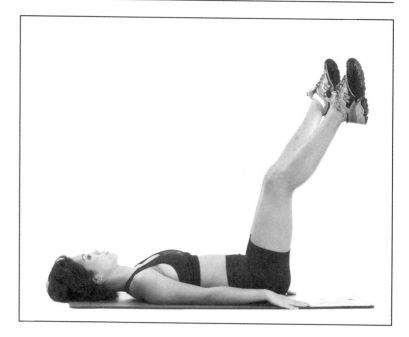

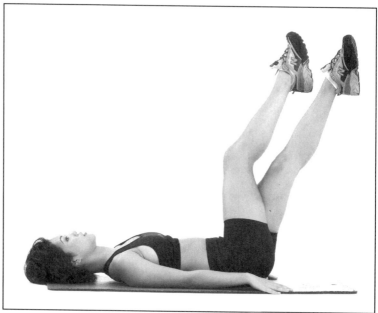

Side Bend

To start:

Stand with your legs shoulder width apart, your knees slightly bent. Draw your navel inward. With one arm, hold a 15 to 20 pound dumbbell. Raise your other arm to shoulder height. Bend it at the elbow, with your fist facing your head.

Instructions:

1. Bend laterally at the waist. Bend to the side that is holding the dumbbell. Contract your obliques hard.

2. As you bend toward one side, straighten your opposite arm, bringing your fist over you head.

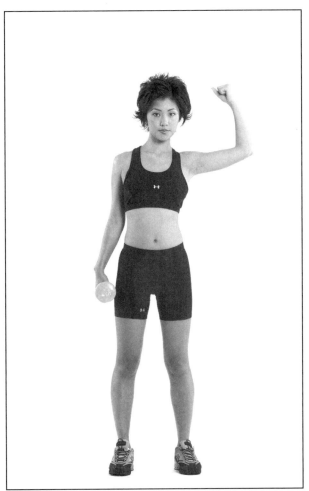
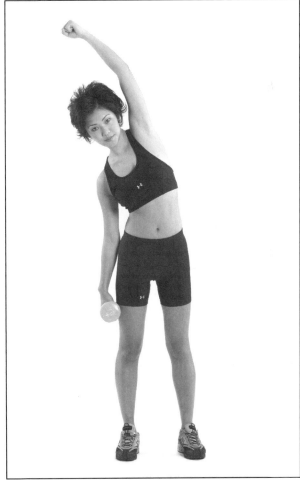

Reverse Crunch with Physioball

To start:

Lie on the floor and place a physioball between your knees, grasping it firmly with your ankles. Place your hands alongside your body.

Instructions:

1. Lift your hips off the floor, contracting your abdominals as the ball touches your chest.
2. Lower slowly under control, and repeat for repetitions.

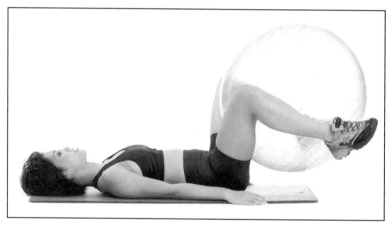

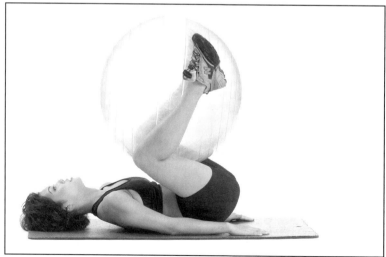

Bent Leg Hip-Raise

To start:

Lie on the floor with your hands at your sides, knees bent and feet flat on the floor.

Instructions:

1. Begin to rotate your hips upward and over, toward your chest.

2. Slowly lower your feet to the starting position.

Note: Do not allow your feet to touch the floor. If you feel pain in your lower back, limit the range of motion by not coming up so high.

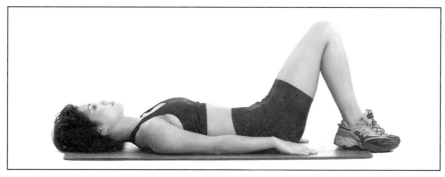

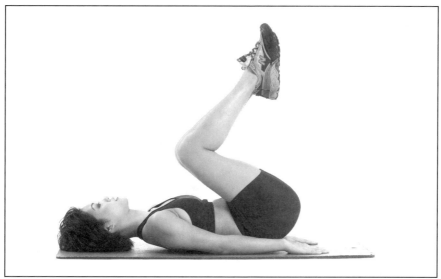

Bicycle

To start:

Lie on the floor with your hands loosely behind your head. Raise your legs to form a 90-degree angle at your knees.

Instructions:

1. As you curl your upper body and crunch your abdominal muscles, bring your left elbow toward your right side while drawing your right knee in to meet it.
2. Continue to alternate sides, back and forth.

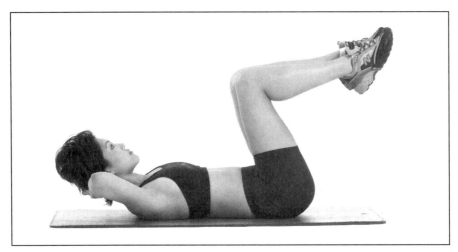

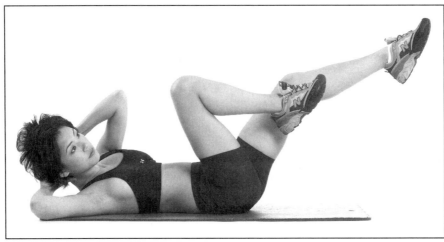

Hands Over Head Crunch

To start:

Lie on your back. Lift your legs off the floor so your knees form a 90-degree angle. Bring your arms over your head to the floor. Press your arms against your ears, and interweave your fingers.

Instructions:

1. Begin to curl your upper body 2 inches off the floor.

2. Contract your abdominal muscles on the way up, bringing your rib cage toward your pelvis.

3. Lower, without letting your head touch the floor. Repeat.

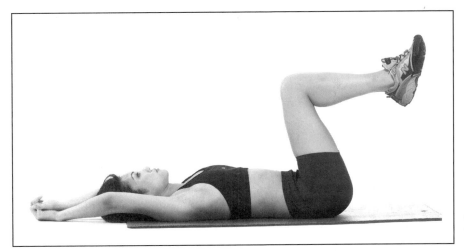

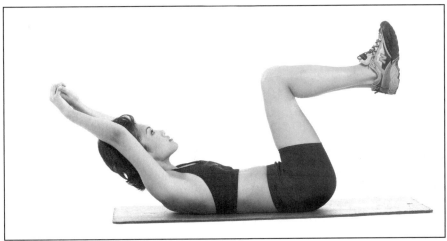

Figure-Four Crunch

To start:

Lie on an exercise mat. Bend your knees to a 90-degree angle. Cross your left leg over your right knee. Your knees should be directly over your hips. Place your hands loosely behind your head. Do not pull on your neck.

Instructions:

1. Contract your abdominal muscles and lift your upper body off the floor while simultaneously lifting your glutes a few inches.

2. Return to the starting position.

3. Repeat for the required number of repetitions, then change legs.

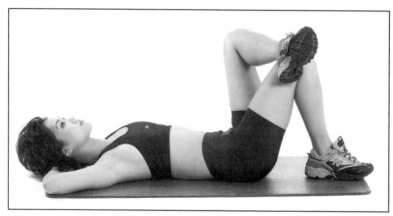

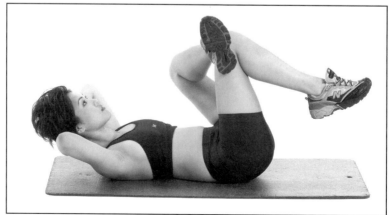

Twisting Crunch on the Physioball

To start:

Sit on top of a physioball. Balance yourself by placing your feet firmly on the floor. Allow the ball to roll until your upper back is centered on top of the ball. Place your hands loosely behind your head.

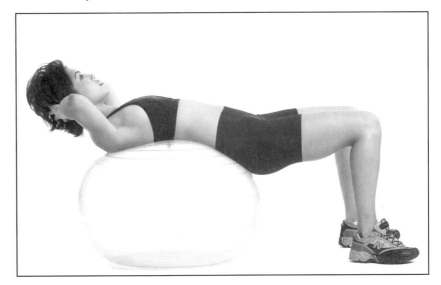

Instructions:

1. Crunch forward and contract your abdominal muscles, rotating your left elbow toward your opposite knee.

2. Return to the starting position, rotating your body back to the original position.

3. Repeat, alternating to the other side after each crunch.

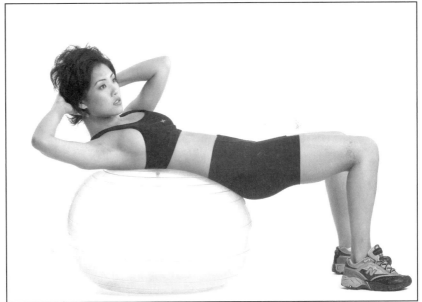

Hip Thrust

To start:

Lie on your back with your arms along the sides of your body. Raise your legs perpendicular to the floor.

Instructions:

1. Contract your abdominal muscles to lift your hips a few inches off the floor.

2. Push your heels toward the ceiling. Do not allow your buttocks to touch the floor.

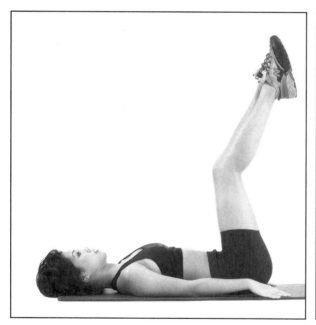 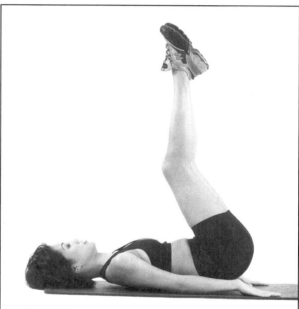

Reverse Crunch

To start:

Lie on your back with your arms by your side, your knees bent, and your feet flat on the floor.

Instructions:

1. Raise your hips off the floor toward your chest.

2. Contract your lower abdominal muscles. Do not allow your feet to touch the floor.

3. Return your hips to the floor with control.

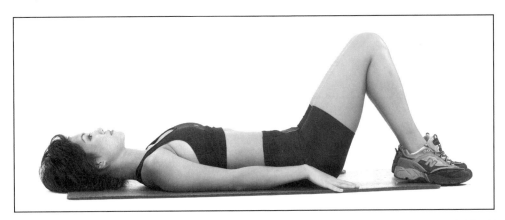

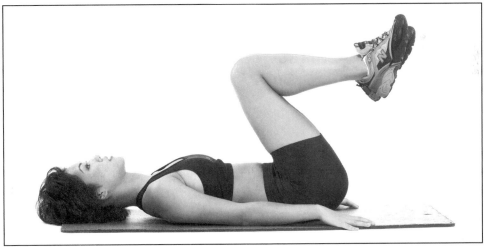

Side Jackknife

To start:

Lie on your right side, placing your arm in a comfortable position. Straighten your legs and place them on top of each other. Place your left hand on your head.

Instructions:

1. Lift your left leg while simultaneously bending your torso up to the side.

2. Contract your oblique muscles as the top of the movement.

3. Slowly lower to the starting position.

Note: Use this as a substitute for the Decline-Bench Twisting Crunch

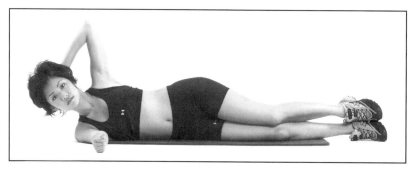

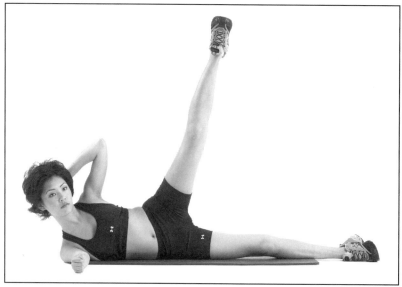

ABDOMINAL EXERCISES FOR THE GYM

Decline Bench Twisting Crunch, 78

Vertical-Bench Leg Raise, 79

Hanging Run-in-Place, 80

Cable Crunch with Rope, 81

Machine Crunch, 82

Hanging Knee Raise to the Side, 83

Reverse Crunch on Incline Board, 84

Decline-Bench Twisting Crunch

To start:

The higher you set the bench angle the more difficult the movement becomes. Select the appropriate angle for you. Secure your feet firmly against the rollers, place your hands over your chest or loosely behind your head.

Instructions:

1. Lie back slowly and lower your body 10 inches away from the bench.
2. Curl back up by twisting your arms to the opposite side knee.
3. Complete all reps on one side, then alternate sides.

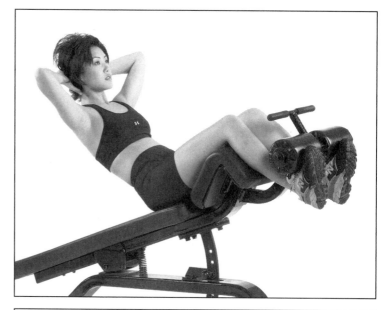

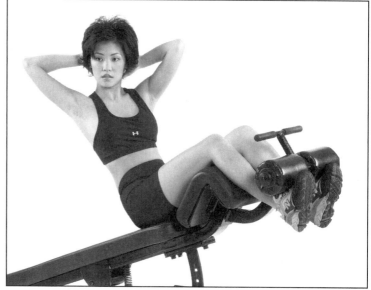

Vertical-Bench Leg Raise

To start:

At the vertical bench, step up onto the foot platform, hold onto the handles, place your back flat against the pad.

Instructions:

1. Rotate your pelvis forward and raise your legs until they are parallel to the floor.

2. Contract your abdominals at the top, then slowly lower your legs and repeat.

3. If this is too difficult, bend your knees to a 90-degree angle, and raise them to chest level.

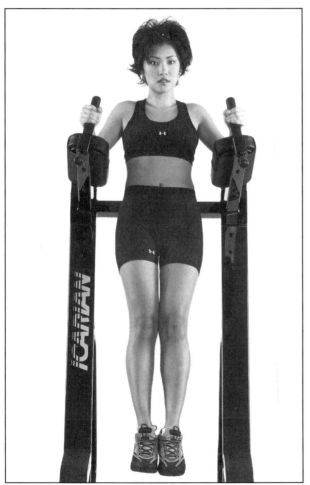
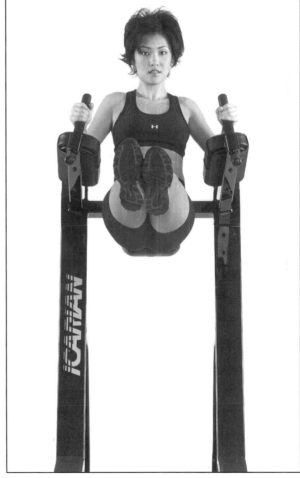

Hanging Run-in-Place

To start:

At the vertical bench, step onto the foot platform, grasp the handles, hold your body up by straightening your arms into a locked position.

Instructions:

1. Bring your knees up toward your abdomen, alternating legs, one at a time, in a slow, controlled motion. Hang, running in place for 20 seconds.

2. Work up to 50 seconds.

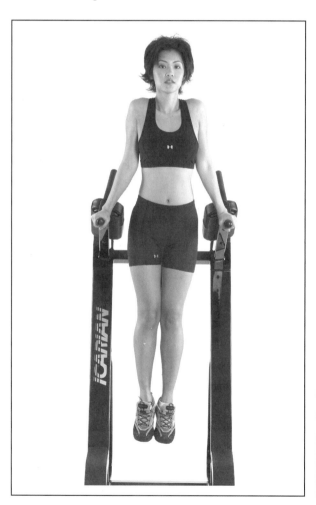
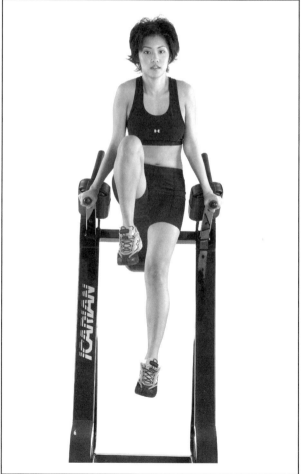

Cable Crunch with Rope

To start:

Attach a rope to the upper cable pulley of the universal machine. Step 2 feet away from the machine and face the weight stack. Kneel on the floor. Grasp the rope attachment and place your arms on both sides of your head, your hands along side your ears.

Instructions:

1. Curl your body forward and down bringing your elbows toward the ground.

2. In a controlled motion crunch your abdominal muscles and return to the top of the movement.

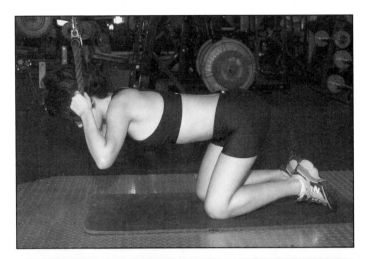

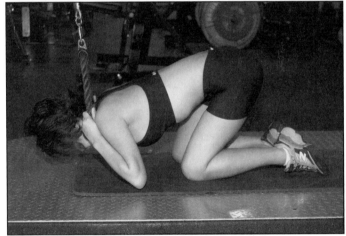

Machine Crunch

To start:

Sit on the crunch machine. Adjust the pad so it rests on the upper part of your chest. Place your feet on the platform so that your knees form a 90-degree angle. Place your arms on the handles in front of your chest for support.

Instructions:

1. Slowly lower the chest pad toward your ribcage and pelvis in a controlled manner.
2. Contract your abdominal muscles and slowly return to the starting position.

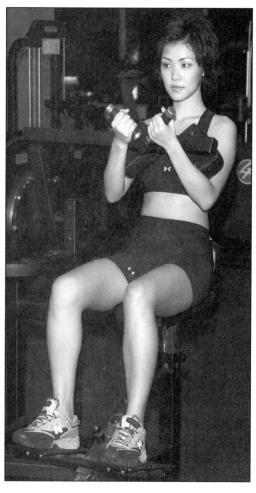
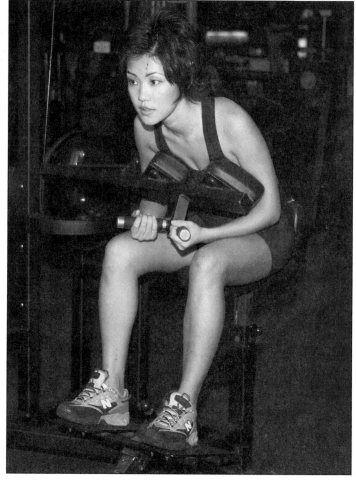

Hanging Knee Raise to the Side

To start:

At the Vertical Bench, step up to the front platform, hold onto the handles, and place your back flat against the pad.

Instructions:

1. Bend at the knees, and without swinging your body, rotate your hips and bring your knees as high as you can to one side.

2. Contract your abdominal muscles and slowly lower your knees.

3. Repeat on the same side before beginning the other side.

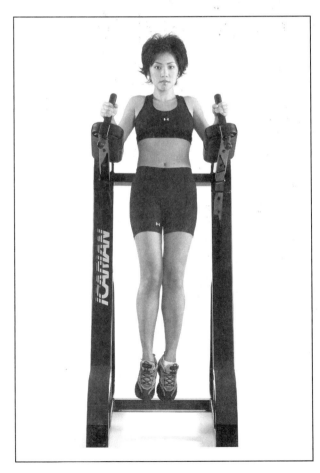
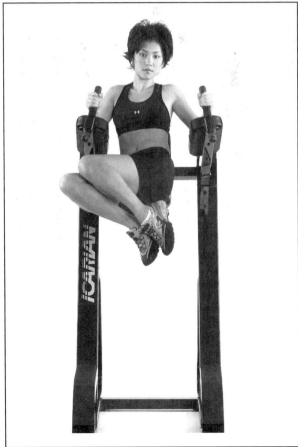

Reverse Crunch on Incline Board

To start:

Lie down on an incline board. The higher the incline the more difficult the movement becomes. Grasp the bench edge with your hands firmly. Keep your legs bent at a 90-degree angle.

Instructions:

1. Rotate your hips and pelvis forward until your knees touch your chest.

2. Slowly, lower your legs.

Note: Stop immediately if you feel pain in your lower back.

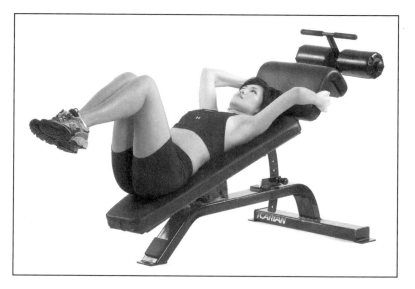

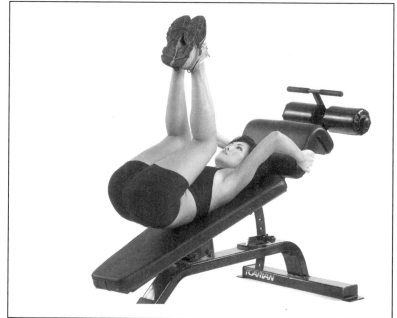

Strength Training Exercises

Strength training builds lean muscle tissue, making the body look tighter and shapelier. It is the only means of increasing muscle tissue. No matter how many aerobics classes you take, it will not shape your body by increasing muscle tissue. If you want your arms to look defined, you must include strength training in your workout.

Strength training significantly increases your metabolic rate through the addition of muscle, which increases the body's need for calories. Strength training burns a substantial four to ten calories per minute, depending on your size and fitness level. There is an important secondary benefit to strength training: your body's fat stores are only burned in muscle tissue, so the more muscle you have, the more fat burning machinery your body maintains.

In the *Bridal Bootcamp*™ workout, you will do strength training for twenty minutes, bringing your heart rate to 65-75 percent of your maximum heart rate.

Here are some tips for making the most of your strength training exercises:

- Wear your heart rate monitor. Before you start set the monitor to show your percentages instead of beats per minute. If you are not at your training zone, pick up the pace.
- Warm up. Remember that your body must be warmed up to loosen up your body and prepare the muscles for lifting.
- Maintain strict form. Stabilize your body so that the primary muscles in the lift do the work.
- Train with maximum intensity. Take every set to failure, which means that you no longer have the ability to complete another set of repetitions in perfect form.
- Maintain consistent tempo. Perform all sets in a slow and controlled manner.
- Rest only up to 40 seconds between sets. Do not allow muscles to fully recover their energy supply between sets. By doing this you increase your effectiveness of your sets as you force your body to adapt to the weight faster.

- Starting weights. Choose a weight that will cause failure at the high number of repetitions during the first set of reps. For example, if you plan to do 3 sets of 15, 12, 10 repetitions each, you should pick a weight that will not enable you to perform more than 15 repetitions.

- Add weights. Continue to force your body to adapt to a greater weight load. You must add more weights when you can perform more than the high number of repetitions in the first set in perfect form. As with the above example, if you can perform more than 15 repetitions in the first set, then the weight originally chosen is now too light. Lift a heavier weight.

- Do not over train. Even if you are having the time of your life, do not train more than 4 days per week with weights and no more than 60 minutes per workout.

- Take a break. After every three-month program, take five days off.

STRENGTH TRAINING EXERCISES IN THE GYM

Leg Press, 89

Bench Dip, 90

Rear Deltoid Flyes, 91

Lying Leg Curl, 92

Leg Press Calf Raise, 93

Seated Calf Raise Machine, 94

Seated Leg Curls, 95

Standing Calf Raise, 96

Seated Cable Rows, 97

Triceps Press Down, 98

One Arm Reverse-Grip Press Down, 99

Two Arm High Cable Curl, 100

Overhead Rope Extension, 101

Cable Crossover, 102

Smith Machine Squats, 103

Smith Machine Reverse Lunges, 104

Leg Extensions, 105

Pec Dec, 106

Preacher Curls, 107

Hack Squat, 108

Barbell Lunges, 109

Flat Dumbbell Press, 110

Standing Barbell Circles, 111

Barbell Squats, 112

Abductor Machine, 113

Adductor Machine, 114

Seated Machine Press, 115

Shoulder Press Machine, 116

Wide Grip Front Pulldown, 117

Lying Tricep Barbell Extension, 118

Assisted Pull-Up Machine, 119

Close Grip Bench Press, 120

Standing Leg Curl, 121

One Arm Preacher Dumbbell Curls, 123

Assisted Push-Ups, 124

Flat Dumbbell Flyes, 125

Dumbbell Concentration Curls, 126

One Arm Dumbbell Rows, 127

Incline Dumbbell Press, 128

Seated Dumbbell Press, 129

Leg Press

Benefits:

This exercise shapes and strengthens the front and back of your thighs and glutes.

To start:

Sit in the leg press machine with your back and hips squarely against the back support. Draw your navel inward. Place your feet shoulder width apart against the platform.

Instructions:

1. Slowly lower the platform towards your body until you reach a 90-degree angle in your knees. Be sure that you do not lower it too close to your chest, creating too much pressure on your lower back.

2. Rapidly press it back to starting position, making sure you do not lock out your knees.

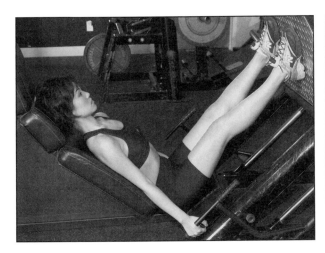 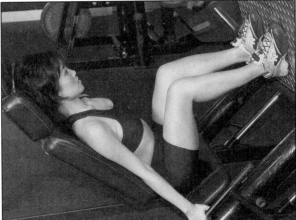

Bench Dip

Benefits:

This exercise shapes and strengthens the back of your arms.

To start:

Sit at the edge of the bench, placing your hands by your hips, fingers at the edge of the bench, elbows pointed to the rear. Draw your navel inward. Hold your body up as you place your feet flat on the floor, knees at a 90-degree angle.

Instructions:

1. Slowly lower your body toward the floor until you feel a stretch in your triceps, the muscle along the back of the arm. Keep your back close to the bench as you descend.

2. Push yourself back up and straighten your arm completely, contracting your triceps at the top of the movement.

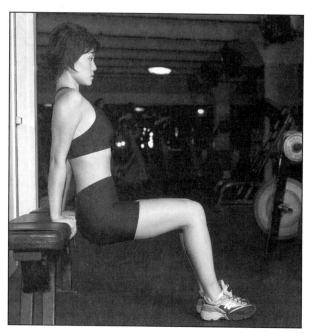 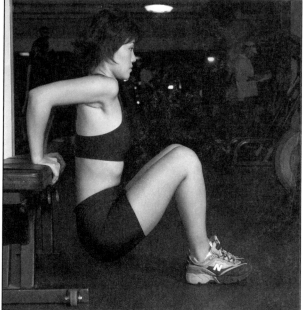

Rear Deltoid Flyes

Benefits:

This exercise shapes and strengthens the back of your shoulders and upper back.

To start:

Sit facing the rear deltoid machine, placing your feet firmly on the floor. Grab onto the machine handles and draw your navel inward.

Instructions:

1. Begin by pulling on the machine handles and extend your arms to your sides.

2. Contract your shoulder and back muscles.

3. Slowly return to the starting position.

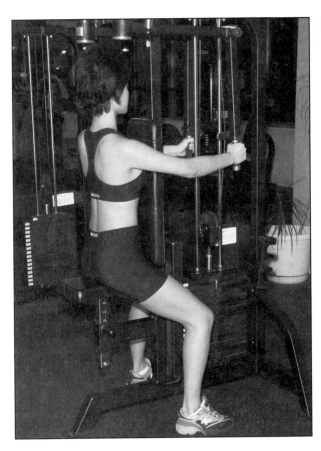 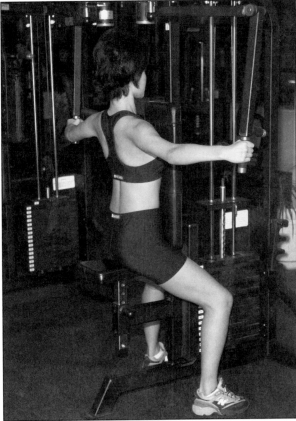

Lying Leg Curl

Benefits:

This exercise strengthens and shapes the back of your thighs.

To start:

Lie face down on the bench. Place your knees beyond the edge of the bench. Adjust the rollers so that they rest on the back a little above your ankles. Hold on to the handles on the side, keeping your gaze straight ahead.

Instructions:

1. Slowly raise and flex your knees to raise your feet against the rollers. Your feet should almost touch your glutes.

2. Lower and return to the starting position.

Note: Make sure that you do not lift your hips off the bench, putting too much pressure on your lower back.

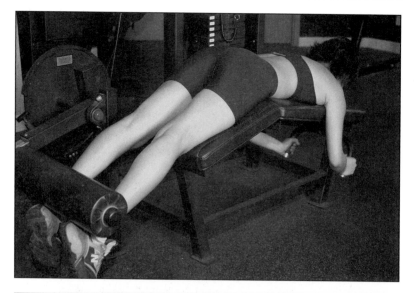

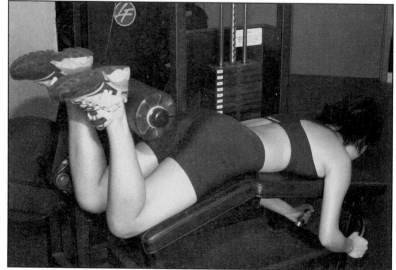

Leg Press Calf Raise

Benefits:

This exercise shapes and strengthens your calves.

To start:

Sit on an incline leg press machine with your lower back in full contact with the pad. Place the balls of your feet at the edge of the foot platform. Keep your toes pointed straight ahead. Do not lock your knees. Grip the machine handles for stability.

Instructions:

1. Slowly lower your heels until your feel a slight stretch.
2. Raise your heels as high as you can and contract your calves.

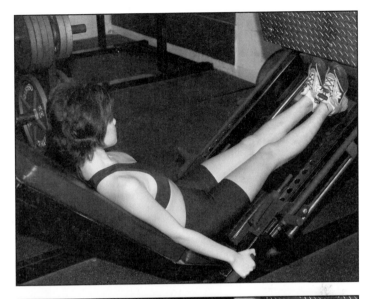

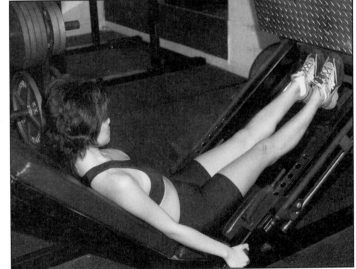

Seated Calf Raise Machine

Benefits:

This exercise shapes and strengthens your calves.

To start:

Sit on the calf raise machine. Adjust pads snuggly over your lower thighs. Maintain a straight back.

Place the balls of your feet firmly on the platform. Keep your toes pointed straight ahead.

Instructions:

1. Raise your heels as high as possible and unlatch the safety bar.

2. Slowly lower your heels with control until they are as far below the balls of your feet as possible.

3. Quickly rise on the balls of your toes and contract your calves at the top of the movement.

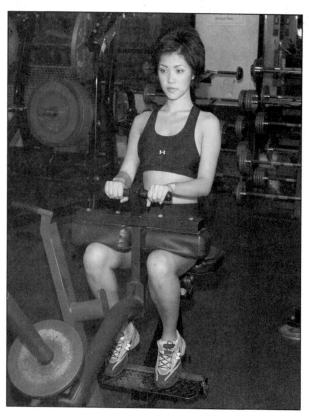 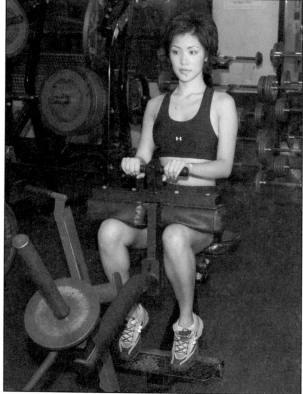

Seated Leg Curls

Benefits:

This exercise strengthens and shapes the back of your legs.

To start:

Sit on the seated leg-curl machine with your back firmly pressed against the pad. Make sure the back rest is adjusted so that your knees clear the edge of the seat. Adjust the leg rollers so that they rest right above your ankles.

Instructions:

1. Keep your feet flexed and begin to contract your hamstrings as you lower both legs down, creating a 90-degree angle in your knees.

2. Hold for two seconds.

3. Slowly return to the starting position.

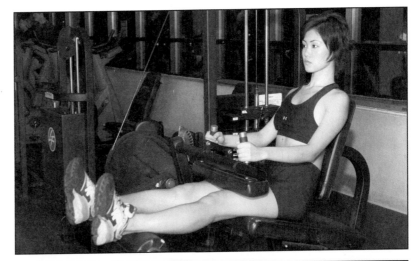

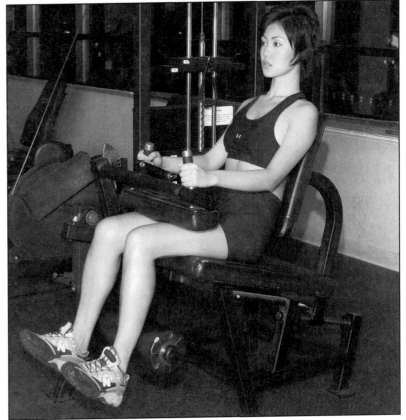

Standing Calf Raise

Benefits:

This exercise shapes and strengthens your calves.

To start:

Stand on the calf-raise machine platform with your shoulders underneath the pads. Grip the handles on the top of the machine for support. Place the balls of your feet firmly on the foot platform with your toes pointing straight ahead. Keep your legs straight and torso erect. Do not lock your knees.

Instructions:

1. Slowly lower your heels until you feel a stretch in your calf muscles.

2. Quickly rise as high as possible on the balls of your feet and contract.

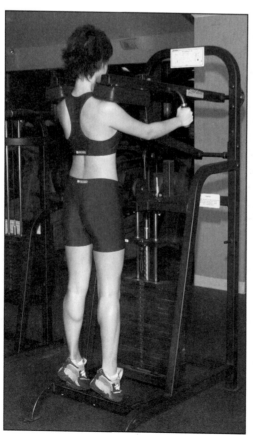 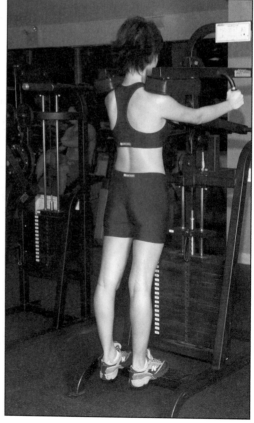

Seated Cable Rows

Benefits:

This exercise strengthens and shapes your back.

To start:

Sit down on seated row bench machine. Draw your navel inward. Keep your back straight. Place your feet on the platform with your legs slightly bent. Choose a handle that has a double neutral grip and attach to the lower pulley cable.

Instructions:

1. Hold the handles and pull them toward your midsection.
2. Pull your shoulder blades together and contract your back muscles.
3. Extend your arms in front of you and lean slightly forward.

Note: Be sure to keep your torso erect.

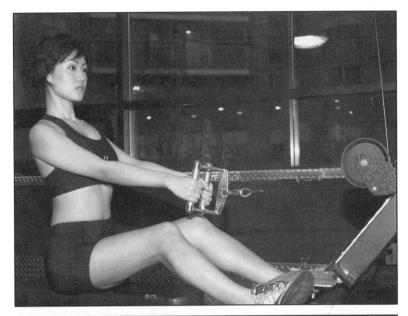

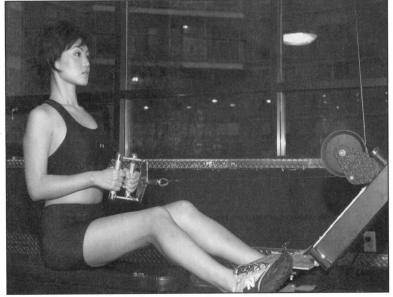

Triceps Pressdown

Benefits:

This exercise shapes and strengthens the back of your arms.

To start:

Stand in front of a high cable machine with your feet shoulder width apart. Draw your navel inward.

Hook a V bar attachment and grab it with a palms-down grip. Keep your elbows at your sides.

Instructions:

1. Press the v bar down with your hands.

2. As you pass the 90-degrees elbow position, straighten your arms out and squeeze your triceps hard.

3. Slowly bring it back up toward your chest.

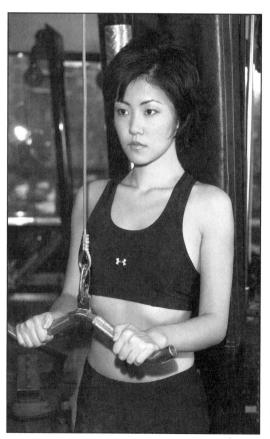 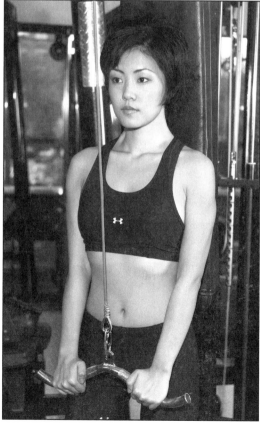

One Arm Reverse-Grip Press Down

Benefits:

This exercise shapes and strengthens the back of your arms.

To start:

Attach a stirrup handle to the upper pulley of a cable station and hold it with a palms-up grip. Stand sideways so that your working arm lines up with the upper pulley cable. Stand with your feet shoulder width apart and with one leg slightly in front of the other. Draw your navel inward. Keep the working elbow firmly against your side.

Instructions:

1. Pull down the handle and straighten your arm completely, contracting your triceps as you move.

2. Hold this position for 2 seconds.

3. Repeat through the first set, and then switch to the other arm.

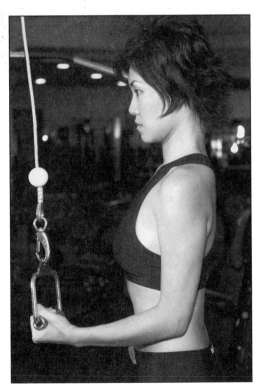 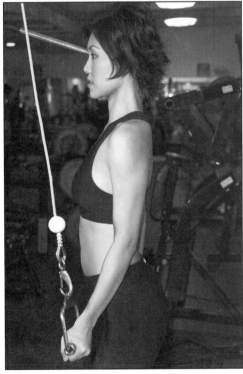

Two Arm High Cable Curl

Benefits:

This exercise strengthens and shapes your biceps.

To start:

Attach a pair of stirrup handles to the upper pulley of a cable station. Grasp the handles with a palms-up grip and stand midway between the two cables. Bring your arms out to your sides, fully extended and level with the ground. Draw your navel inward.

Instructions:

1. Keeping your upper arms still, pull the handles toward your head, contracting your biceps hard.

2. Slowly return to the starting position.

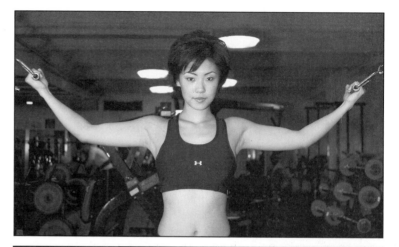

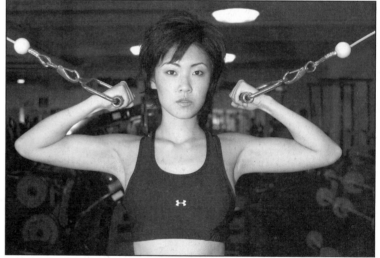

Overhead Rope Extension

Benefits:

This exercise shapes and strengthens the back of your arms.

To start:

Secure the rope attachment to the upper pulley of a cable station. Grasp the rope attachment with a neutral grip. Turn your body so that the weight stack is behind you and raise your arms overhead. Your elbows should be bent and the rope behind your head. Draw your navel in. Your feet should be parallel, or one foot slightly in front of the other. Bend slightly at the waist, maintaining a straight back.

To start:

1. Begin by extending you arm straight out in front of your body. Tightly contract your triceps.
2. Slowly return to the starting position.

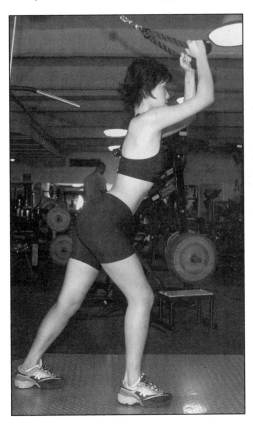 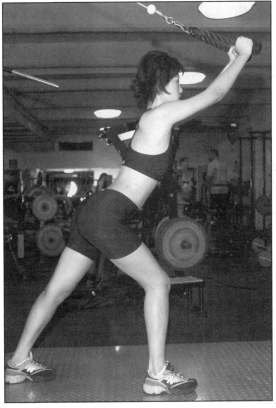

Cable Crossover

Benefits:

This exercise shapes and strengthens your chest.

To start:

Attach a pair of stirrup handles to the upper pulleys of a cable station. Grasp the handles with a palms down grip. Step slightly in front and away from the pulleys. Keep your feet shoulder width apart and your arms in line with the cables. Bend forward at the waist about 30 degrees, maintaining a straight back. Draw your navel inward.

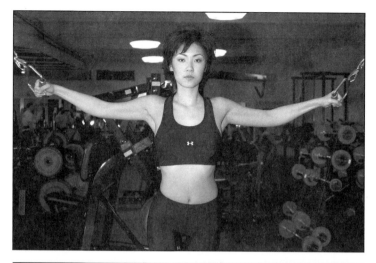

Instructions:

1. Keep your elbows slightly bent and draw your arms together in front of your body, contracting your chest muscles as you do so.

2. Release the contraction slowly and return to starting position.

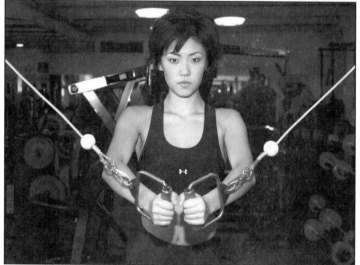

Smith Machine Squats

Benefits:

This exercise shapes and strengthens the front and back of your thighs and tightens your glutes.

To start:

Stand under the bar of the Smith Machine with your feet shoulder width apart. Draw your navel inward. Rest the bar high on your shoulders. Your hips should be directly under your shoulders. Keep your torso erect.

Instructions:

1. Lower your body until your thighs are parallel to the floor, forming 90-degree angles in your knees.
2. Push up with your legs and press the bar up. Do not lock your knees.

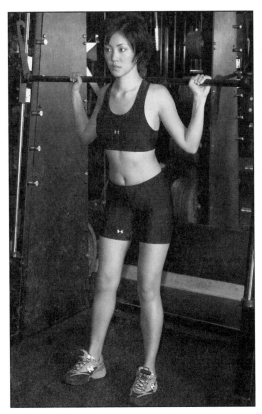 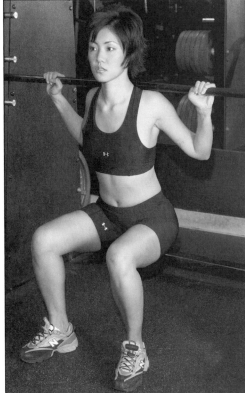

Smith Machine Reverse Lunges

Benefits:

This exercise shapes and strengthens the front and back of your thighs and tightens your glutes.

To start:

Stand under the bar of the Smith Machine with your feet pointed straight ahead, Draw your navel inward. Hold the barbell with your hands wider than shoulder width apart. Release the safety lever.

Instructions:

1. Begin bending the knee of your forward leg for greater support and stability as you take a medium step to the rear with your torso erect. Your knees should form a right angle directly above your toes.

2. Do not allow the back knee to touch the floor. As you lunge backward, you should feel tension in the front leg, specifically the quadriceps. As you step back to the starting position, you should feel tension in your glutes on that side of the body.

3. Repeat through the first set, and then switch to the other leg.

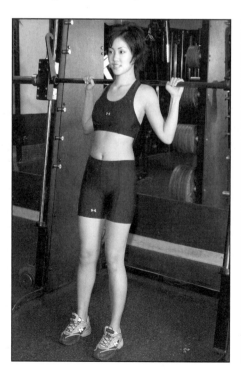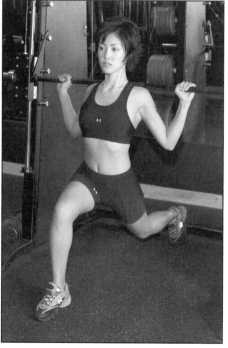

Leg Extensions

Benefits:

This exercise shapes and strengthens the front of your thighs.

To start:

Sit on the leg extension machine seat with your back firmly pressed against the pad. Draw your navel inward. Adjust the rollers so that they press against your shins. Keep your feet flexed. Grasp the handles alongside the seat.

Instructions:

1. Straighten your legs slowly to their full extension and hold for 2 seconds. Do not lock your knees.

2. Lower them to the starting position.

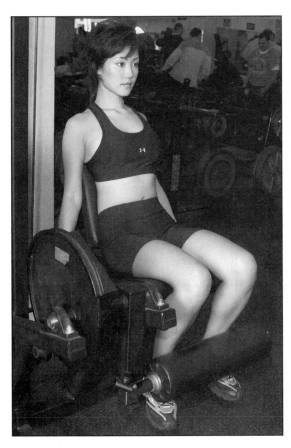 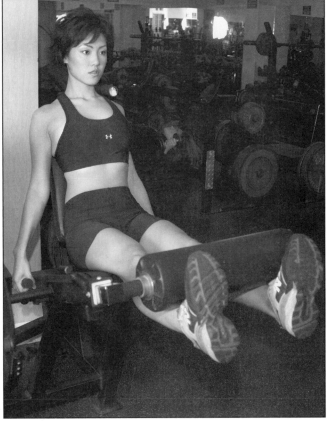

Pec Dec

Benefits:

This exercise shapes and strengthen your chest.

To start:

Adjust the seat of the machine so that your arms are in line with your shoulders. Sit with your torso erect against the back pad. Place your forearms against the resistance pads. Draw your navel inward.

Instructions:

1. Push the resistance pads toward each other and contract your chest muscles hard at the top of the movement.

2. Slowly return your arms to start until your elbows are in line with your shoulders.

Note: Make sure your shoulders maintain full contact with the backpad.

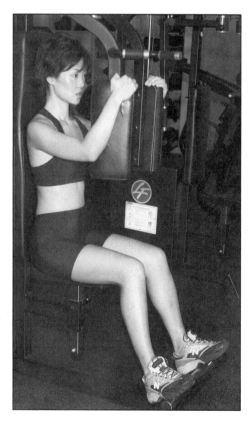 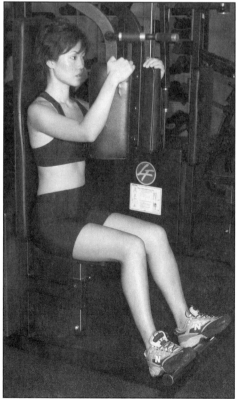

Preacher Curls

Benefits:

This exercise shapes and strengthens your arms.

To start:

Sit down at the Preacher Curl Machine. Place the back of your upper arms against the incline support pad. Sit in an erect position. Draw your navel inward.

Instructions:

1. With your upper arm firmly against the pad, grab the handles on the bar and begin curling your arms up toward your face.

2. Squeeze your biceps at the top of the movement.

3. Slowly lower to the starting position.

4. Repeat through the first set, and then switch to the other arm.

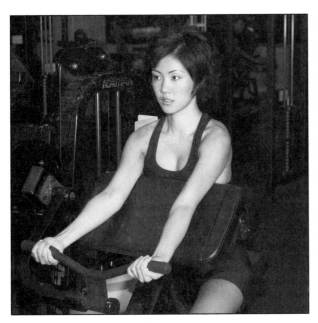 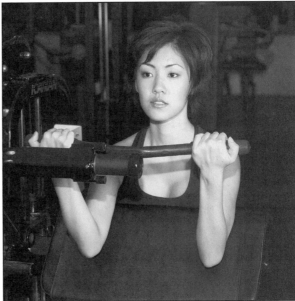

Hack Squat

Benefits:

This exercise shapes and strengthens the front and back of your thighs and tightens your glutes.

To start:

Position yourself on the Hack Squat Machine so the resistance pads rest on your shoulders. Keep your back firmly against the pad and draw your navel inward. Place your feet shoulder width apart against the platform. Release the safety levers.

Instructions:

1. Lower your body into a squat position until your thighs are about parallel to the platform. There should be 90-degree angle in your knees.

2. Rapidly press it back to starting position. Do not lock your knees.

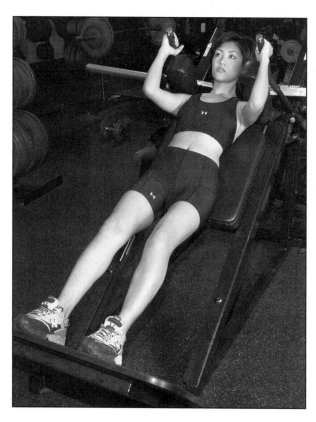
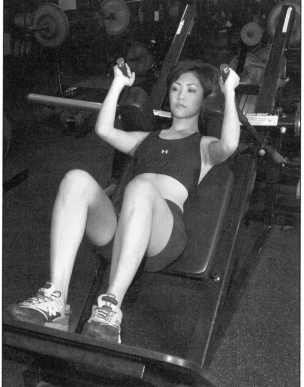

Barbell Lunges

Benefits:

This exercise shapes and strengthens the front and back of your leg and tightens your glutes.

To start:

Grab a barbell with your hands wider than shoulder width apart. Place the barbell behind your neck, and draw navel inward.

Instructions:

1. Step forward with one leg. As your foot lands, bend both knees to lower your body. Your front knee should form a right angle directly above your toes. Keep your torso erect.

2. Stand back up by pressing through your front foot. Bring both legs together.

3. Repeat through the first set, then switch to the other leg.

Note: Do not allow the back knee to touch the floor. As you lunge forward with your front legs, you should also feel tension in your quadriceps, and as you step back you should feel tension in your glutes.

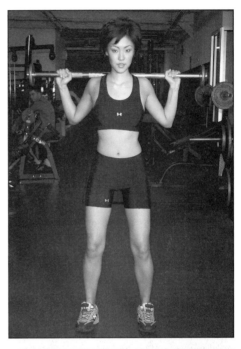

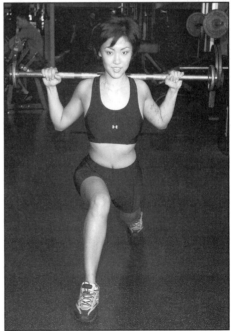

Flat Dumbbell Press

Benefits:

This exercise shapes and strengthens your chest.

To start:

Lie face up on an exercise bench. Make sure your feet are flat on the floor, knees bent 90 degrees. Hold a pair of 5- or 10-pound dumbbells with a palms-up grip. Extend your arms fully so that the weights are directly above your chest, almost touching each other.

Instructions:

1. Lower the weights so that your elbows point out from your sides and the dumbbells are in line with your chest.

2. Push the dumbbells back up, contracting your chest muscle to the start position.

Note: For the at-home workout, lay over a physioball to do this exercise.

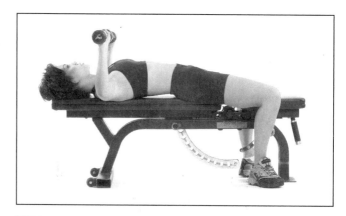

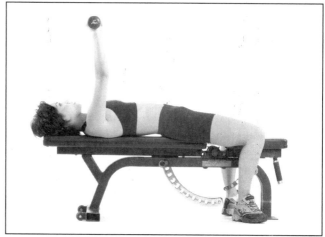

Standing Barbell Curls

Benefits:

This exercise shapes and strengthens your arms.

To start:

Stand with your feet shoulder width apart. Draw your navel inward. Hold a barbell with both hands at about shoulder width with a palms-up grip. Extend your arms in front of your thighs. Keep your elbows along the sides of your body.

Instructions:

1. Curl the barbell up toward your chest in a slow, controlled motion, contracting your biceps at the top.

2. Lower the bar slowly. Do not allow the bar to rest on your thighs.

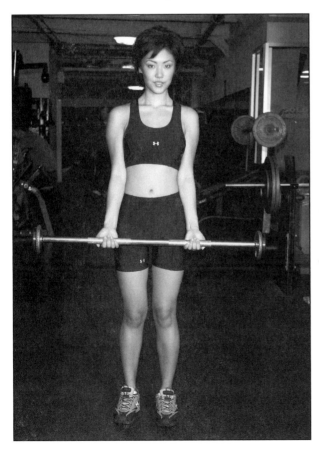 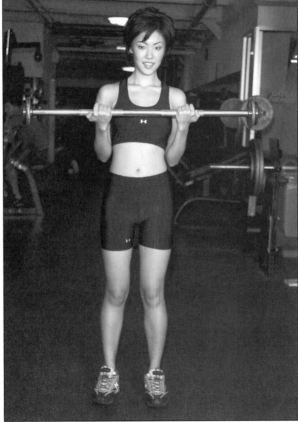

Barbell Squats

Benefits:

This exercise shapes and strengthens the front and back of your thighs and tightens your glutes.

To start:

Stand in front of a mirror. Grab a barbell. Let it rest high on your shoulders. Draw your navel inward. Your hips should be directly under your shoulders. Maintain a straight torso.

Instructions:

1. Lower your body until your thighs are parallel to the floor, forming 90-degree angles in your knees and hips.

2. Push up with your legs and press the bar up. Do not lock your knees.

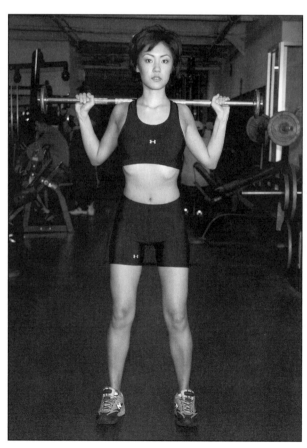 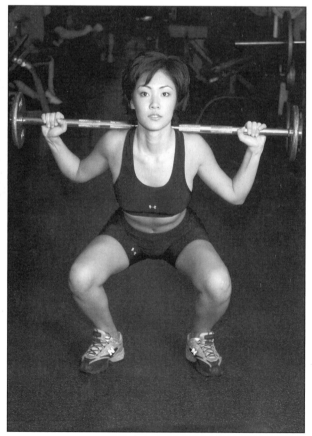

Abductor Machine

Benefits:

This exercise shapes, strengthens, and tightens the outside of your thighs.

To start:

Sit erect at the adductor machine. Place your thighs against the resistance pads and secure your feet firmly on the footrest. Draw your navel inward.

Instructions:

1. Begin to separate your thighs, pressing your knees against the resistance pads.

2. Hold for two seconds, and slowly return to the stating positions. Do not allow the weight stack to touch together.

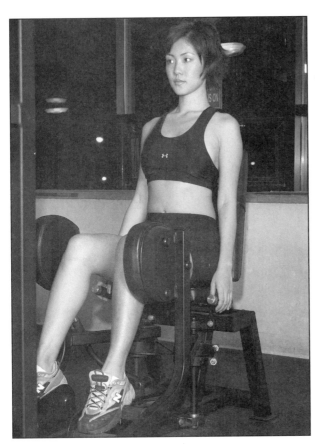 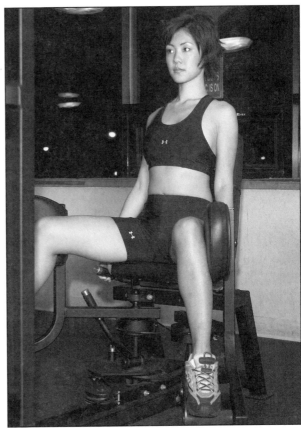

Adductor Machine

Benefits:

This exercise shapes and strengthens the inside of your thighs.

To start:

Sit erect at the adductor machine. Place your thighs against the resistance pads and secure your feet firmly on the footrest. Draw your navel inward.

Instructions:

1. Draw your thighs together, pressing your knees against the resistance pads.

2. Hold for two seconds, and slowly return to the starting position. Do not allow the weight stack to touch together.

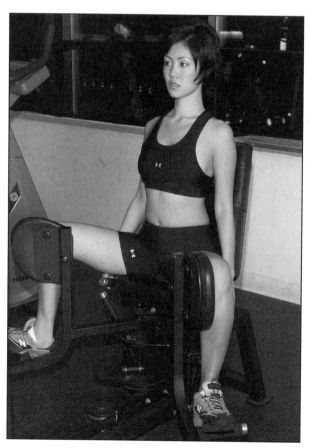 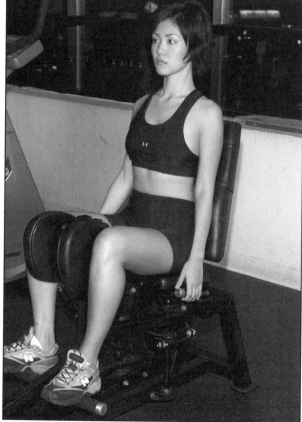

Seated Chest Press Machine

Benefits:

This exercise shapes and strengthens your chest.

To start:

Sit on the seated press machine, with your back firmly against the pad, your feet flat on the floor. Draw your navel inward. Adjust the seat so that machine handles are in line with your upper chest. Grasp the handles with a palms-up grip.

Instructions:

1. Push against the machine handles and extend your arm in front of you, contracting your chest muscles. Hold for 2 seconds.

2. Slowly lower the handles back to the starting position without letting the weight stack touch.

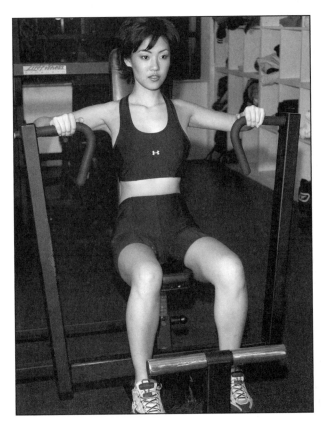 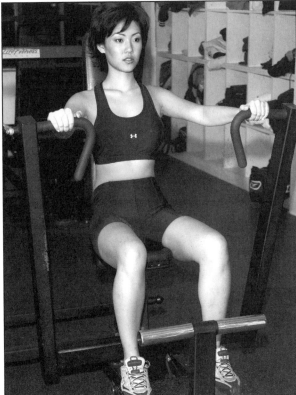

Shoulder Press Machine

Benefits:

This exercise shapes and strengthen your shoulders.

To start:

Sit on the shoulder press machine, adjusting the seat to the appropriate height. Keep your feet firmly on the ground. Draw your navel inward. Grab on to the machine handles with a palms-up grip. Pinch your shoulder blades against the pad.

Instructions:

1. Begin by pressing the machine handles up by extending your arm fully. Do not lock your elbows.

2. Slowly lower your arms so that your elbows form a 90-degree angle.

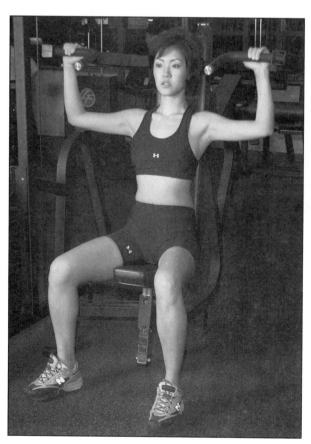 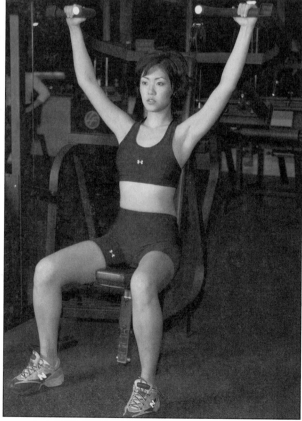

Wide Grip Front Pulldown

Benefits:

This exercise shapes and strengthen your upper back.

To start:

Sit at the lateral pull down machine. Adjust the knee pads so that they fit snugly over your thighs. Place your feet flat on the floor. Draw your navel inward. Keep your torso erect. Grasp the bar with a palms-up grip.

Instructions:

1. Draw your shoulder blades together and pull the bar down toward your chest, just past your chin.
2. Hold this position for 2 seconds.
3. Slowly straighten your arms, bringing the bar overhead.

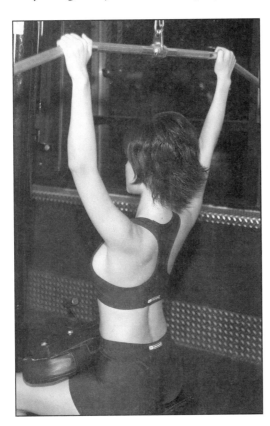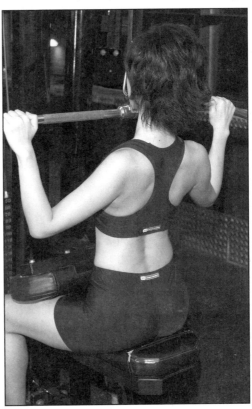

Lying Tricep Barbell Extension

Benefits:

This exercise strengthens and shapes the back of your arms.

To start:

Lie on a flat bench with your feet flat on the floor. Have a spotter hand you an EZ-bar and grasp it with a palms-up grip. Extend your arms above your chest, then lower them to a 45-degree angle toward your head.

Instructions:

1. Keeping your upper arms in place, lower the bar until it is 2 inches above your forehead.

2. Raise the bar by straightening your arms fully, contracting your triceps as you come back to the starting position.

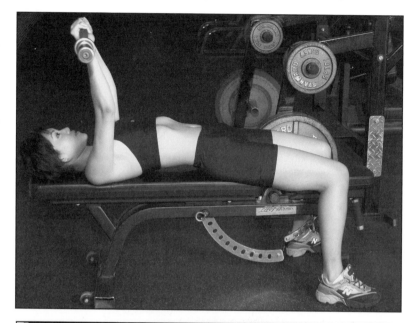

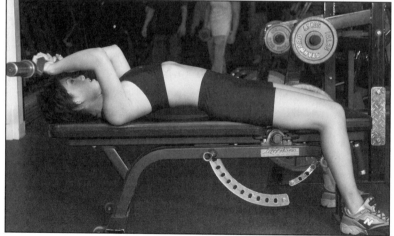

Assisted Pull-Up Machine

Benefits:

This exercise shapes and strengthens your back.

To start:

Step up to the elevated platform. Grab the overhead bar with a palms-up grip that is slightly wider than shoulder width apart. Extend your arms and relax your shoulders to fully stretch your back. Draw your navel inward.

Instructions:

1. Pull yourself up until your chin is even with the bar.

2. Contract your back at the top of the movement.

3. Slowly lower to the starting position.

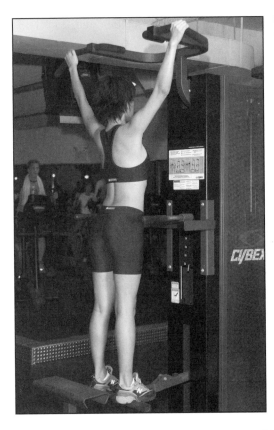 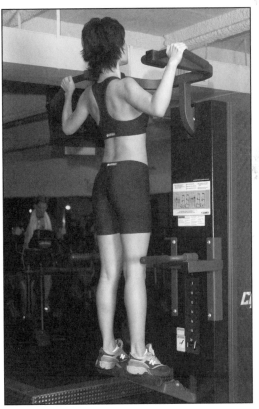

Close Grip Bench Press

Benefits:

This exercise shapes and strengthens the back of your arms.

To start:

Grab a 20 or 30-pound pre-weight set barbell. Lie down on an exercise bench. Keep a slight arch in your lower back. Take a palms facing away grip on the bar with your hands closer than shoulder width apart. Press the bar up and lock your arms.

Instructions:

1. Begin to slowly lower the bar down to your chest. As the bar gets close to your chest begin to press the bar back up, squeezing your triceps muscles.

2. Repeat for repetitions

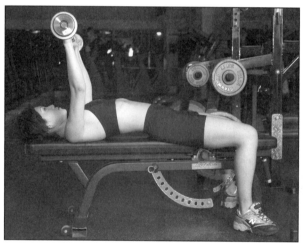 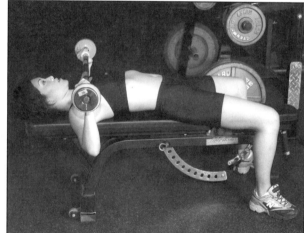

Standing Leg Curl

Benefits:

This exercise shapes and strengthens the back of your thighs.

To start:

Stand in front of a leg curl machine. Keep your torso upright. Place the back of one ankle against the resistance roller. The front of the working leg should rest against the front pad at all times. Hold the machine handles. Draw your navel inward.

Instructions:

1. Flex your foot, and begin to bend your knee without letting the pad touch your glutes.

2. Lower the resistance pad slowly, with control.

3. Repeat the required number of repetitions.

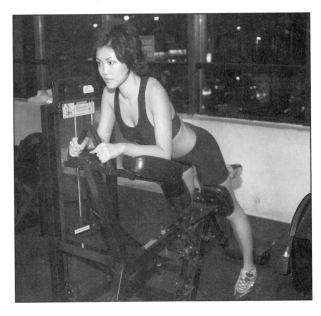
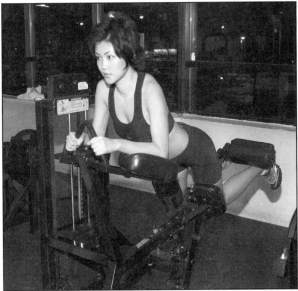

STRENGTH TRAINING MISCONCEPTIONS

Most women have preconceived notions about strength training. Once you do strength training consistently, you'll see that most of your assumptions are not true.

Myth 1: "I Don't Want To Get Too Big."

Your wedding workout is meant to destroy fatty tissue, and as an adaptive measure your body rebuilds bigger and stronger. More important, women never build muscles like men can for one reason: testosterone. Women have $1/20$ the testosterone of men, therefore no matter what they do, they will not build muscle the way a man does. If you exercise hard and lift heavy weights you will only build lean muscle and harden your body. And that's what we are here for, right?

Myth 2: "I Only Need Aerobics."

If you do lots of cardiovascular training, you will burn body fat, but you will also burn muscle tissue. The result is an unhealthy thin, yet flabby body. It's true that aerobic activity does burn calories. But an hour after you finish exercising, the increase in calorie burning stops and your body returns to normal. However, if you gain 5 pounds of muscle, it will help you burn about 200 calories more a day, without doing any further exercise. Remember the key to metabolism is lean muscle.

Myth 3: "The Rest of Me Is Fine, I Just Want To Flatten My Stomach."

Most women do not want to strength train their entire body, instead they just want to rid of some body fat in a specific area. But there's no such thing as spot reducing. Nor is it possible to tone fat. Our genetic make up determines where we carry body fat.

Myth 4: "If I Stop Exercising, All My Hard Work Will Turn Into Fat."

Muscle is muscle and fat is fat. One cannot convert into the other. Lack of exercise is often followed by poor eating habits, which results in weight gain.

One Arm Preacher Dumbbell Curls

Benefits:

This exercise shapes and strengthens your arms.

To start:

Grab a dumbbell with a palms up grip. Place the back of your upper arms against an incline support pad. Sit in an erect position. Draw your navel inward.

Instructions:

1. With your upper arm firmly against the pad, curl the dumbbell up, squeezing your biceps at the top of the movement.

2. Slowly lower the dumbbell.

3. Repeat through the first set, and then switch to the other arm.

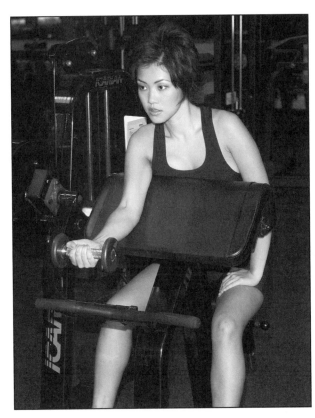 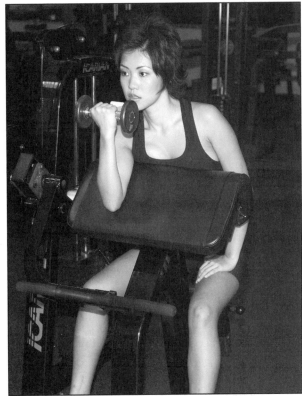

Assisted Push-Ups

Benefits:

This exercise will shape and strengthen your chest, shoulders, biceps, and triceps.

To start:

Place your arms a little more than shoulder-width apart on the bench. Keep your back flat and your neck in alignment with your spine.

Instructions:

1. Bend your elbows and slowly lower your chest a few inches above the bench.

2. Press down into your palms and begin to raise your chest up.

Note: If you are doing the at-home workout, use the edge of a windowsill or your kitchen table.

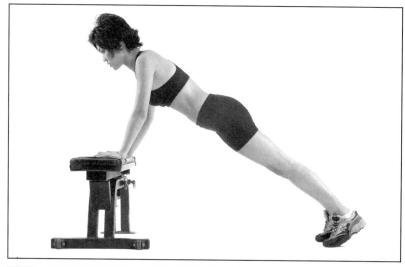

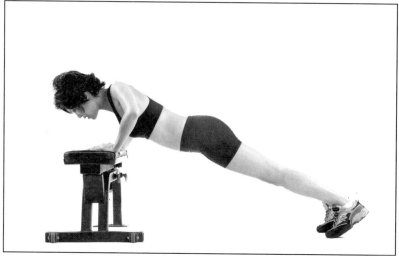

Flat Dumbbell Flyes

Benefits:

This exercise shapes and strengthens your chest.

To start:

Lie down on an exercise bench with your feet flat on the floor. draw your navel inward. Grab a pair of 5- or 10-pound dumbbells with palms facing each other. Extend your arms above your chest, elbows slightly bent. Pinch your shoulder blades against the pad.

Instructions:

1. Lower your arms out to your sides to about shoulder level.
2. Begin to contract your chest muscles to bring your arms together, forming an arc with your arms.

Note: For the at-home workout, lie over a physioball to do this exercise.

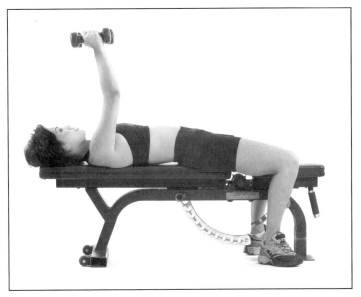

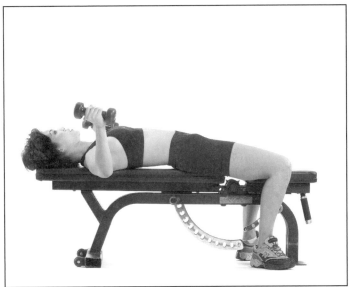

Dumbbell Concentration Curls

Benefits:

This exercise shapes and strengthens your arms.

To start:

Sit at the edge of an exercise bench. Draw your navel inward. Keep your legs apart and feet flat on the floor. Grab a 10-pound dumbbell and lean forward. Let your free arm hang to the side of your thighs, but do not lean on your leg.

Instructions:

1. Raise the dumbbell straight up toward your shoulder. Do not rest at the top of the movement.

2. Contract your biceps and slowly lower to the starting position. Do not stop at the top of the movement. Keep constant tension on the muscle.

Note: For the at-home workout, perform this exercise while sitting on a physioball or a chair.

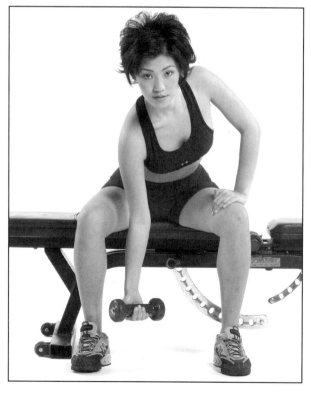 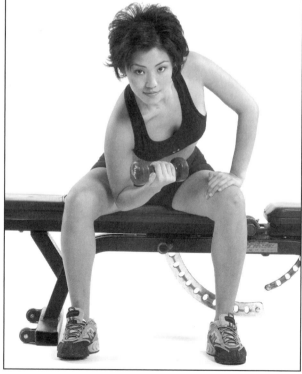

One Arm Dumbbell Rows

Benefits:

This exercise shapes and strengthens your back.

To start:

Place your right hand and your right knee on an exercise bench. With your left hand, grasp a 10- or 15-pound dumbbell, with a neutral grip. Allow the working arm to hang straight down. Draw your navel inward. Maintain a flat back and look ahead.

Instructions:

1. Pull the dumbbell upward toward your chest.
2. As the elbow passes the shoulder, contract your back muscles.
3. Lower to the starting position.

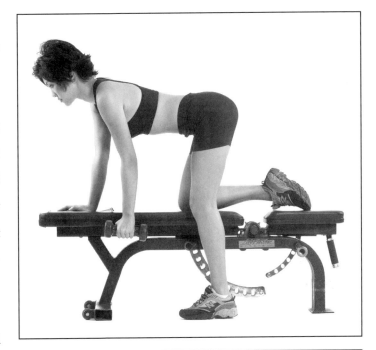

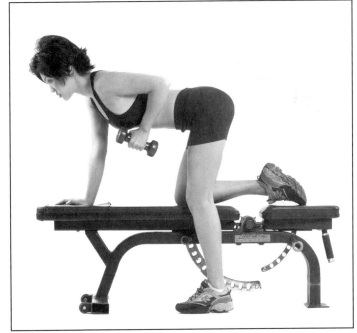

127

Incline Dumbbell Press

Benefits:

This exercise shapes and strengthens your chest.

To start:

Lie on an incline bench set at approximately a 30- to 45-degree angle. Keep your feet flat on the floor and draw your navel inward. Grab a pair of 5- or 10-pound dumbbells, with a palms-down grip.

Instructions:

1. Extend your arms fully so the dumbbells are directly above your chest almost touching each other. Pinch your shoulder blades against the pad.

2. Slowly lower the dumbbell to shoulder level. Your elbows should form a 90-degree angle.

3. Press the dumbbell upward, using your pectoral muscle. Straighten your arms fully and squeeze at the top.

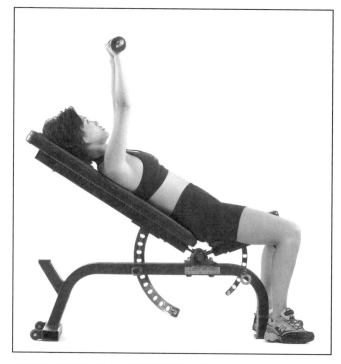

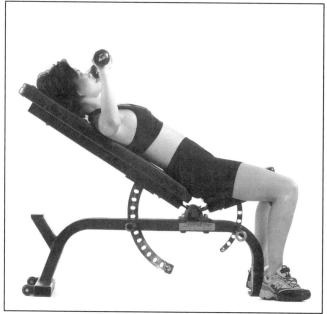

Seated Dumbbell Press

Benefits:

This exercise shapes and strengthens your shoulders.

To start:

Sit on an exercise bench or physioball. Place your feet flat on the floor.

Instructions:

1. Grab a pair of 5- or 10-pound dumbbells, with a palm-down grip. Draw your navel inward.

2. Begin by pressing the dumbbells up, fully extending your arms. Do not lock your elbows.

3. Slowly lower your arms so your elbows form a 90-degree angle.

4. Repeat for the required number of repetitions.

Note: If you are doing the at-home workout, use a chair or physioball to do this exercise.

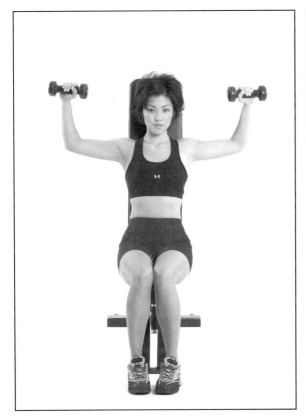 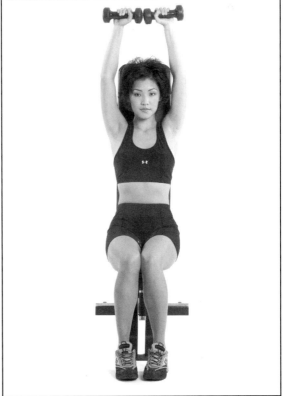

STRENGTH TRAINING EXERCISES YOU CAN DO AT HOME

Bent-Over Lateral Raise, 131

Physioball Dumbbell Squats, 132

Stiff-Leg Deadlift, 133

Physioball One Arm Dumbell Extensions, 134

Standing One Leg Calf Raise, 135

Bent Over Dumbbell Rows, 136

Good Mornings, 137

Front Dumbbell Raise, 138

Chair Dip, 139

Standing Dumbbell Curls, 140

Dumbbell Squats, 141

Alternating Dumbbell Lunges, 142

Overhead Lateral Raise, 143

Upright Rows, 144

Alternating Front Dumbell Raise, 145

Standing Dumbbell Kickbacks, 146

Side Lateral Dumbbell Raise, 147

Leg Lifts, 148

Glute Lifts with Physioball, 149

Physioballl Push-Ups, 150

Hammer Curls, 151

Dumbbell Shrugs, 152

Seated Overhead Dumbbell Extension, 153

Bent-Over Lateral Raise

Benefits:

This exercise shapes and strengthens the rear part of your shoulders and upper back.

To start:

Stand erect, grab a pair of 5- or 10-pound dumbbells with your palms facing each other. Bend at the waist, keeping your back straight and perpendicular to the floor. Draw your navel inward. Keep your knees slightly bent. There should be a slight arch in your lower back. Extend your arms and look forward.

Instructions:

1. Begin by raising your arms straight out to each side, no higher than shoulder level.

2. Contract your rear shoulder muscles and return to the starting position.

Note: Keep your arms in line with your shoulders.

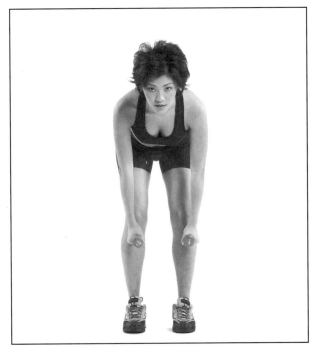 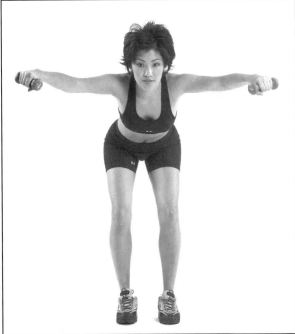

Physioball Dumbbell Squats

Benefits:

This exercise shapes and strengthens the front of your thighs and tightens your glutes.

To start:

Place a pair of 15-pound dumbbells on the floor at your sides. Set a large physioball against a stable wall and stand with your back against it.

Instructions:

1. Roll the ball down the wall as you move into a squat position.
2. Lift the dumbbells off the floor.
3. Stand up with the dumbbells in your hands, and contract your buttocks at the top of the motion.
4. Slowly lower so that your thighs are parallel to the floor. Contract your glutes as you rise back to the starting position.

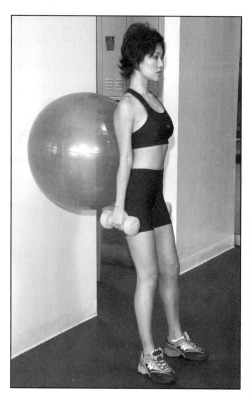
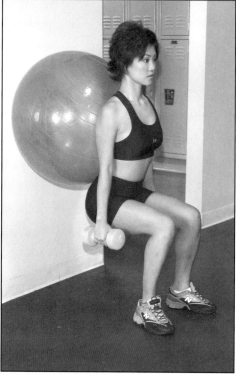

Stiff-Leg Deadlift

Benefits:

This exercise strengthens your lower back and tightens your hamstrings and glutes.

To start:

Stand with your legs shoulder width apart. Draw your navel inward. Grab a pair of dumbbells with palm-down grip. Keep a slight bend in the knees.

Instructions:

1. Slowly lean forward from your hips and lower the barbell down to your shins.

2. Keep your back straight and hold for 1 second and return to the starting position.

Note: If you begin to flex your spine as you lean forward, stop the movement immediately.

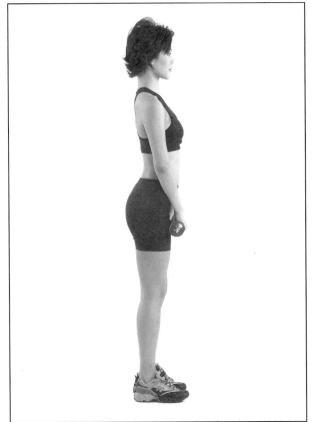 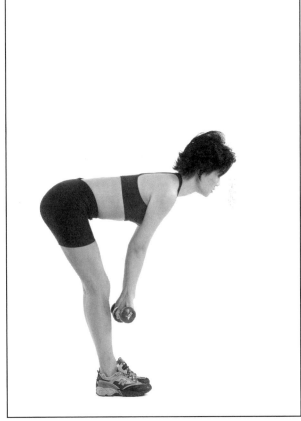

Physioball One Arm Dumbbell Extensions

Benefits:

This exercise shapes and strengthens the back of your arms.

To start:

Grab a 5- or 10-pound dumbbell. Sit on a physioball with your torso erect, feet flat on the floor. Draw your navel inward.

Instructions:

1. Hold the dumbbell with either hand.

2. Bend your arm at the elbow and raise your arm overheard. Keep your arm close to you head.

3. Lower the hand holding the dumbbell behind your head. Your elbows should be pointing up.

4. Keeping your upper arm stationary, press the dumbbell upward until your arm is fully extended.

5. Squeeze your triceps hard.

6. Then switch to the other hand.

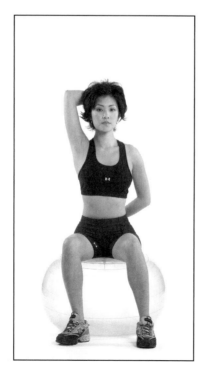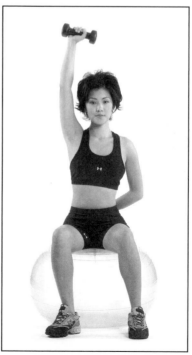

Standing One Leg Calf Raise

Benefits:

This exercise shapes and strengthen your calves.

To starts:

Hold onto a stable chair with one hand. With your other hand, grab a 10- or 15-pound dumbbell.

Raise the leg closest to the chair and rest the ankle behind the standing leg. Draw your navel inward.

Instructions:

1. Rise as high as possible on the balls of your feet. Contract your calve muscles.

2. Slowly lower your legs down to the floor. Repeat for the required number of repetitions, then switch and do the opposite leg.

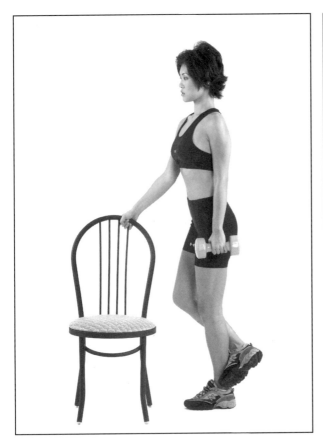 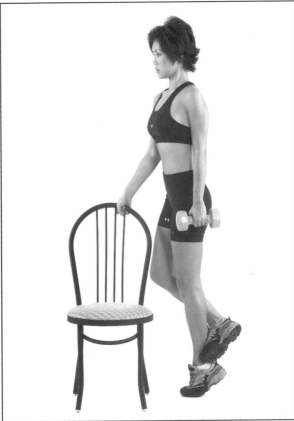

Bent-Over Dumbbell Rows

Benefits:

This exercise shapes and strengthens the middle part of your back.

To start:

Stand upright, holding a pair of 15-pound dumbbells with a palm-up grip. Keeping your back straight, bend forward at the waist. Draw your navel inward. Keep your knees slightly bent. Extend your arms straight and look forward.

Instructions:

1. Pull the dumbbells toward your chest. Keep your elbows close to your sides and concentrate on pulling with your back muscles while you raise your elbows as high as possible.

2. Slowly lower your arms to the starting position.

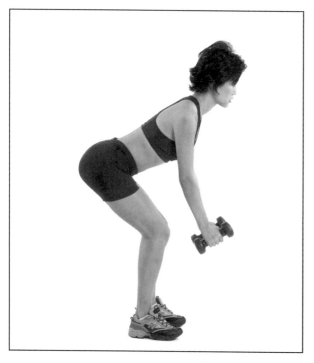 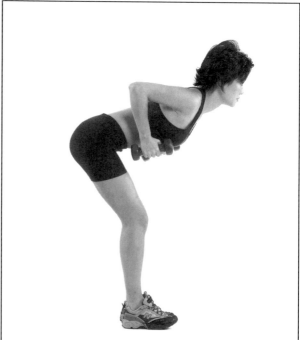

Good Mornings

Benefits:

This exercise shapes and strengthens your lower back, hamstrings, and glutes.

To start:

Stand upright with your feet shoulder width apart. Grab a body bar and place it on your shoulders. Bend your knees slightly, and draw your navel inward.

Instructions:

1. Begin to lean forward from your hips.

2. Rotate your hips backward as your upper body folds forward. Your upper body should be parallel to the floor.

3. In a slow and controlled manner, squeeze your glutes hard as you raise yourself to the starting position.

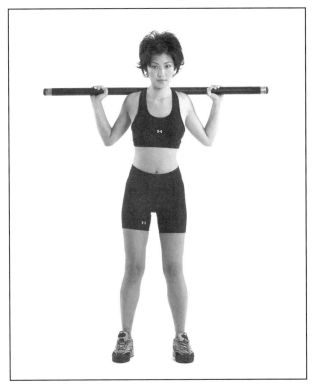
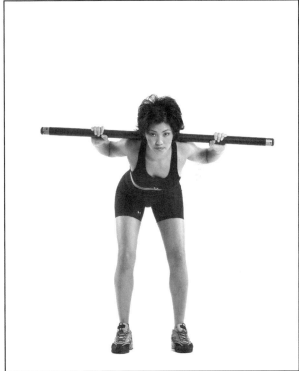

Front Dumbbell Raise

Benefits:

This exercise shapes and strengthens your shoulders.

To start:

Stand erect with you feet shoulder width apart. Draw your navel inward. Grab a pair of 5- or 10-pound dumbbells with a palms-down grip. Extend your arms straight down and in front of your thighs.

Instructions:

1. Raise your arms out in front of you to about shoulder level. Keep your elbows slightly bent.

2. Slowly lower the dumbbells back to the starting position.

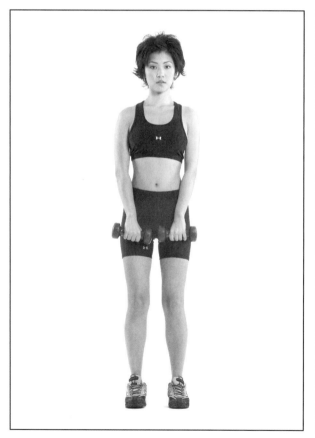 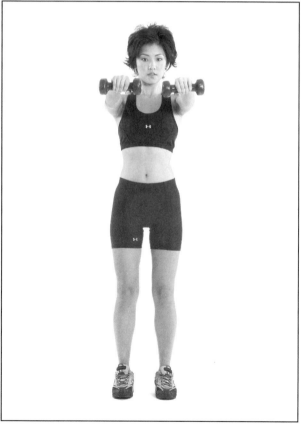

Chair Dip

Benefits:

This exercise shapes and strengthens the back of your arms.

To start:

Sit on the edge of a chair. Place your hands by your hips, fingers cupping the front edge of the chair and your elbows pointing back. Place your feet flat on the floor, knees bent at a 90-degree angle.

Instructions:

1. Bend your elbows to slowly lower your upper body toward the floor. After reaching the bottom position, push yourself upward until your arms are fully extended.

2. Squeeze at the top position.

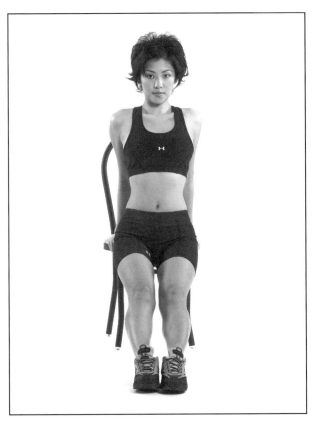
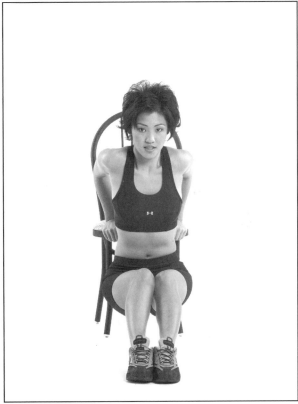

Standing Dumbbell Curls

Benefits:

This exercise shapes and strengthens your arms.

To start:

Stand with your feet shoulder width apart, draw your navel inward. Grab a pair of 5- or 10-pound dumbbells and hold them shoulder width apart with a palms-up grip. Extend your arms in front of your thighs.

Instructions:

1. Curl the dumbbells up, both arms at a time, toward your chest in a slow controlled manner.

2. Contract your biceps at the top of the movement.

3. Lower the dumbbells slowly. Do not allow the bar to rest on your thighs.

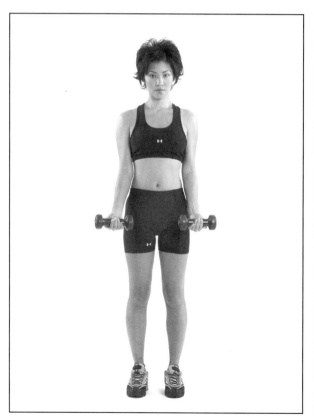
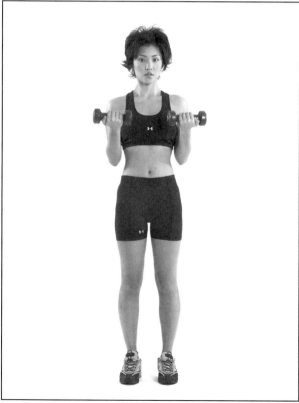

Dumbbell Squats

Benefits:

This exercise shapes and strengthens the front and of your thighs and tightens your glutes.

To start:

Stand with your feet shoulder width apart and grab a pair of 15-pound dumbbells. Draw your navel inward.

Instructions:

1. Lower your body until your thighs are parallel to the floor, forming 90-degree angles in your knees and hips.
2. Slowly raise yourself to the starting position.

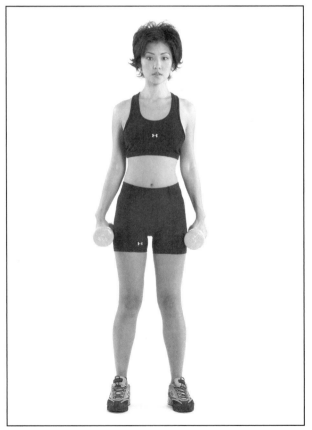
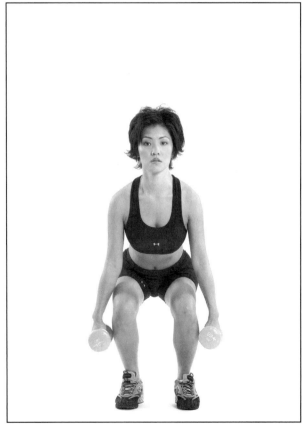

Alternating Dumbbell Lunges

Benefits:

This exercise shapes and strengthens the front and back your thigh and tightens your glutes.

To start:

Stand with your feet about hip-width apart, grab a pair of 15-pound dumbbells and extend your arms out to your side.

Instructions:

1. Take a wide step forward. The front leg and rear leg should form right angles at the knee joint.

2. On the return push, forward from the rear leg to keep the weight on the front leg, and rise to the starting position.

3. Repeat on the other side.

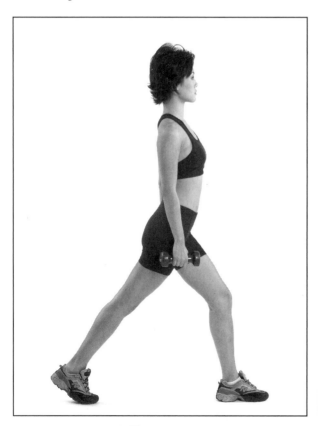 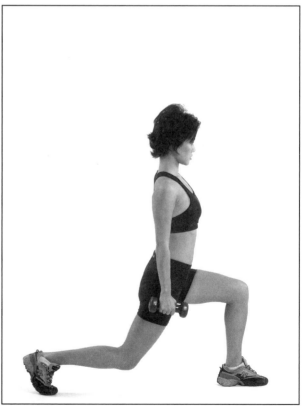

Overhead Lateral Raise

Benefits:

This exercise shapes and strengthens your shoulders.

To start:

Stand erect with your feet shoulder width apart, keeping your abdominal muscles tight. Hold a pair of 5-pound dumbbells and rest them alongside your body.

Instructions:

1. Raise your arms out to the sides and up to a completely overhead position, keeping your elbows slightly bent. Your arms will rotate as you approach the level position.

2. Slowly lower under control.

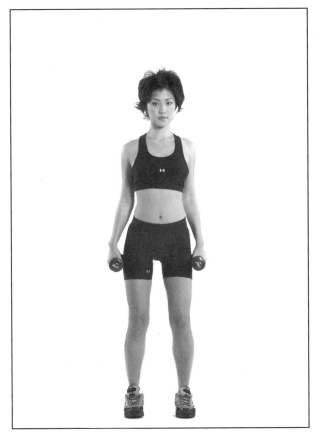 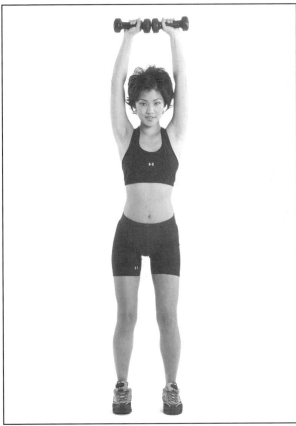

Upright Rows

Benefits:

This exercise will shape and strengthen the sides of your shoulders and upper part of your back.

To start:

Stand with your torso erect. Draw your navel inward. Grab a pair of dumbbells with both hands, using a palms-down grip. Rest your arms in front of your thighs. Your hands should be slightly closer than shoulder width apart.

Instructions:

1. Pull the dumbbells straight up, using the strength in your elbows, not your hands.

2. Raise your arms until they are a little above chest level. Keep the dumbbells six inches in front of your body.

3. Slowly return to the starting position.

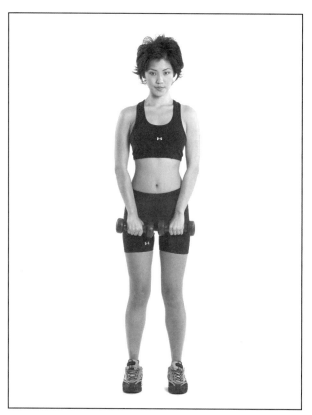 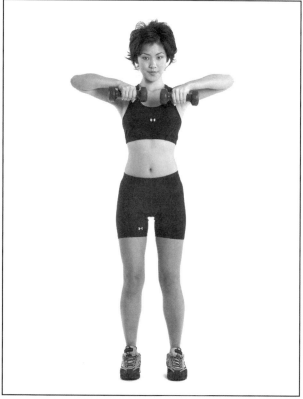

Alternating Front Dumbbell Raise

Benefits:

This exercise shapes and strengthen the front of your shoulders.

To start:

Stand with you feet shoulder width apart. Grab a pair of 5- or 10-pound dumbbells with a palms-down grip. Arms are extended in the front of your thighs.

Instructions:

1. Raise one arm directly in front of your body until you reach shoulder level.

2. Slowly return to the staring position.

3. Alternate sides.

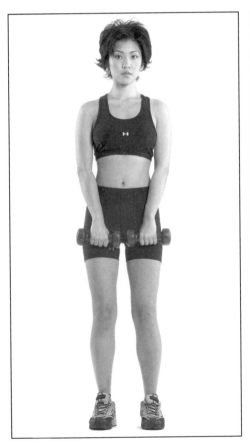 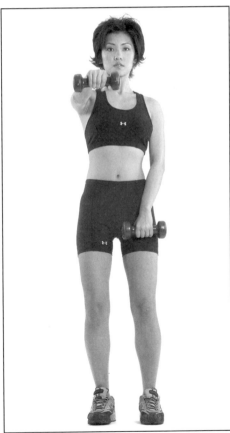

Standing Dumbbell Kickback

Benefits:

This exercise shapes and strengthens the back of your arms.

To start:

Stand with your feet shoulder width apart. Grab a pair of 5-pound dumbbells. Bend at the waist, so your upper body is not quite parallel to the floor. Your knees should be slightly bent with your back straight.

Instructions:

1. Keeping your upper arms alongside your body, bending your elbows at a 90-degree angle.

2. Slowly extend your arms and contract your triceps at the top of the movement.

3. Return to the starting position.

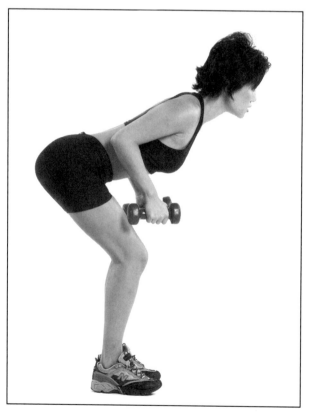
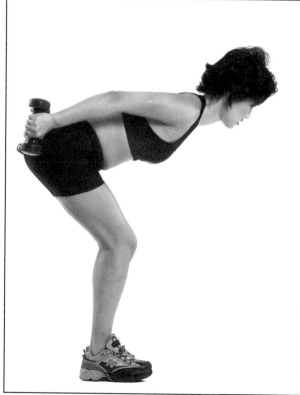

Side Lateral Dumbbell Raise

Benefits:

This exercise shapes and strengthens the sides of your shoulders.

To start:

Stand erect with you feet closer than shoulder width apart, draw your navel inward. Grab a pair of 5-pound dumbbells with a palm-down grip.

Instructions:

1. Extend your arms out to your sides to shoulder level. Keep your elbows slightly bent. Hold for 2 seconds.

2. Slowly lower to the starting position.

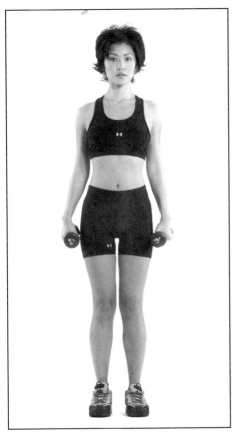 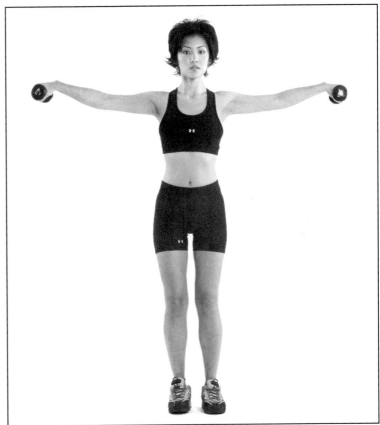

Leg Lifts

Benefits:

This exercise shapes and strengthens your outer thighs.

To start:

Lie on your right side and bend your right leg . Your left leg should be straight out, with your foot rotated in. Support your head with your right arm and stabilize your body by placing the other hand on the floor in front of your body.

Instructions:

1. Lift your left leg as high as you can while maintaining your body in a straight line.

2. Slowly lower your leg in a controlled manner to the starting position.

3. Continue until you have completed the required number of repetitions.

4. Change positions and repeat on the other side.

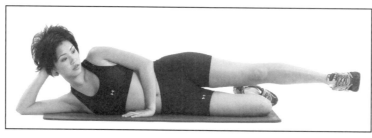

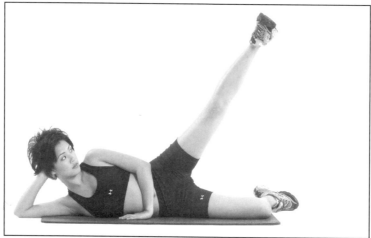

Glute Lifts with Physioball

Benefit:

This exercise strengthens and tightens your glutes.

To start:

Lie down on your back on an exercise mat. Place your heels on the physioball, with your feet a little closer than shoulder width apart. Place your arms along your sides.

Instructions:

1. Lifting your pelvis toward the ceiling, squeeze your glute muscles together. Lift until your back is straight. Do not arch your back.
2. Return to the starting position.

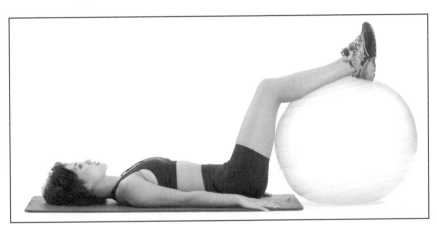

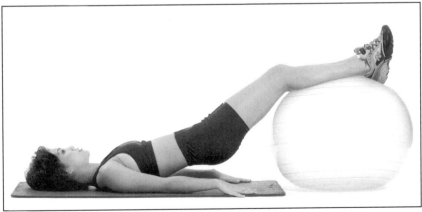

Physioball Push-Ups

Benefits:

This exercise shapes and strengthens your arms, chest and shoulders.

To start:

Lie face down over a physioball. Roll the ball down and balance it under your shins. Place your hands shoulder width apart on the floor. Your body will form a table top. Draw your navel inward, as tight as you can to stabilize your midsection.

Instructions:

1. Begin to bend your elbows and slowly lower your chest to the floor in a push up position.
2. Return to the starting position in a controlled manner.

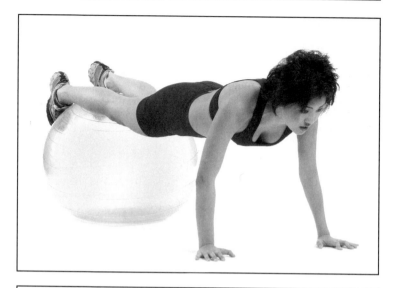

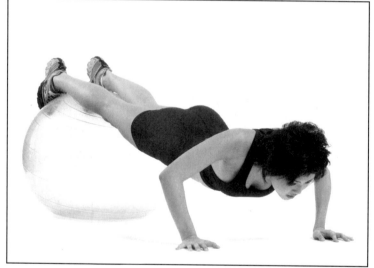

Hammer Curls

Benefits:

This exercise shapes and strengthens your arms.

To start:

Stand upright with your feet shoulder width apart. Draw your navel inward. Grab a pair of 5- or 10-pound dumbbells. Keep your elbows tucked alongside your body during the entire set.

Instructions:

1. Begin by raising the dumbbells toward your shoulders. Contract your biceps at the top of the movement.

2. Slowly lower the weight back down to the starting position.

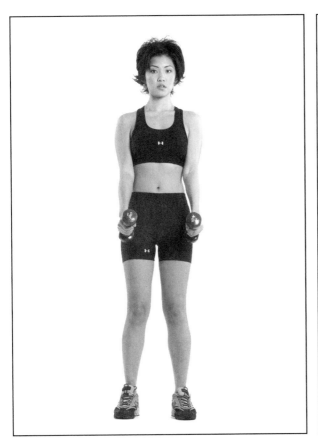 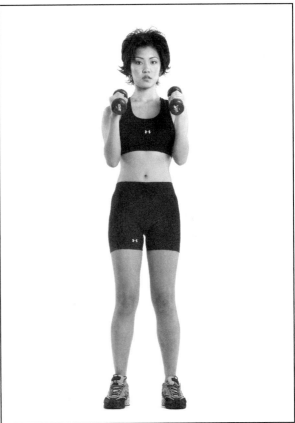

Dumbbell Shrugs

Benefits:

This exercise shapes and strengthens your shoulders and the upper part of your back.

To start:

Grab a pair of 15-pound dumbbells. Stand with your feet shoulder width apart. Draw your navel inward. Place the dumbbells along the outside of your thighs.

Instructions:

1. Raise your shoulders as high as you can and hold for 2 seconds.

2. Slowly lower to the starting position.

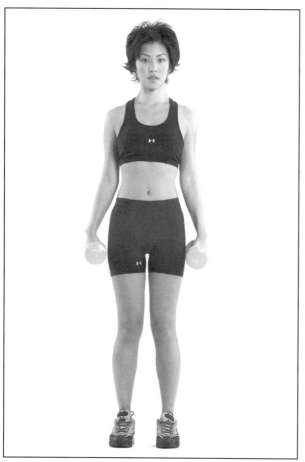 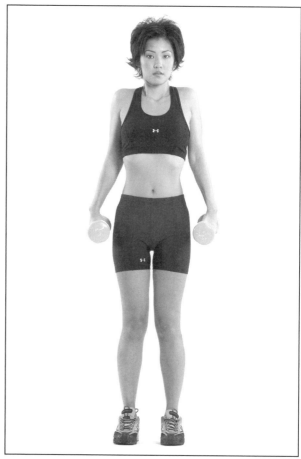

Seated Overhead Dumbbell Extension

Benefits:

This exercise shapes and strengthens your arms.

To start:

Sit on the edge of a chair with your feet flat on the floor, back straight, with both hands, grab a 10- or 15-pound dumbbell. Draw your navel inward.

Instructions:

1. Bend your elbow and raise your arms overhead. Keep your arms close to your ears and the dumbbell behind your head.

2. Keeping your upper arms stationary, lower the dumbbell behind your head, until your elbows form a 90-degree angle.

3. Press the dumbbell upward until your arms are fully extended and contract your triceps

4. Repeat for the required number of repetitions.

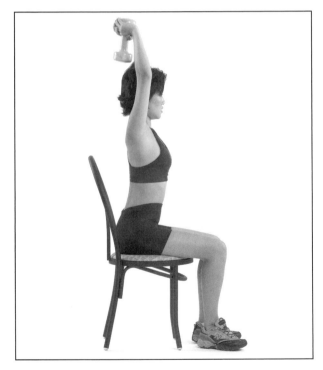 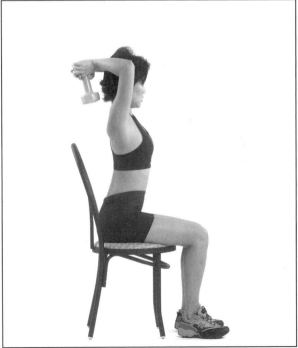

Cardiovascular Exercises

Cardiovascular workouts can help you lose body fat. But if you do not know the correct techniques or use the appropriate equipment, you can end up burning muscle along with fat. If you do it the proper way, then you can get all of the definition you desire and still keep your muscles in great shape. In the chapters ahead, I will show you how to do cardiovascular workouts the right way.

Each of the workouts I have designed for you require twenty minutes of cardiovascular exercise, in which you aim to increase your heart rate to 75 to 80 percent of your maximum heart rate.

You will find a different cardiovascular workout for the six-month, three-month, and one-month workout program:

- For the six-month program, for instance, you will choose one machine to use for a month. If you don't belong to a gym, you can substitute an activity like bicycling or jogging.
- For the three-month program, you'll choose two pieces of equipment for each week.
- For the one-month program, you'll use only one piece of equipment—but not one you used during the three-month workout.

Because each of these workouts differ, I will hold off on the details until you get to the section of the book that covers them.

Post-Workout Cool-Down

Flexibility is as important a component in the fitness equation as strength and endurance. Most sports medicine practitioners believe that increased flexibility reduces the chance of injury; it seems that looser muscles and tendons can withstand greater ranges of motion without tearing. For post workout purposes, static stretching is recommended. Instead of dynamic stretching, where you moved through total joint motion, this time you will hold a position for at least thirty seconds. You want to bring your heart rate down to 50 percent of your maximum heart rate. The program requires five minutes of stretching, specifying which stretches you need.

COOL-DOWN STRETCHES FOR THE SIX-MONTHS PROGRAM

Chest

To start:

You will need a clean, hand towel to complete this stretch. Stand erect with your feet placed shoulder width apart. Tightly hold your towel horizontally at each end.

Instructions:

1. Raise the towel above your head.

2. Slowly bring the towel behind your back, even with your shoulder blades.

3. Pull until you feel the stretch across your chest, and hold the position for at least 30 seconds.

Shoulders

To start:

Sit up straight on the edge of a chair.

Instructions:

1. Lift your shoulders up to your ears, then rotate your shoulders behind your back.

2. Complete the circle by lowering your shoulders downward and then forward.

3. Roll your shoulders in the other direction.

Back: Folded Leaf Posture

To start:

Kneel on the floor with your hands in your lap.

Instructions:

1. Lean forward resting your torso on your thighs, with your forehead resting on the floor, arms extended by your sides, palms facing upward, toes pointed.

2. Hold the position for at least 30 seconds.

Neck

To start:

Sit up straight on the edge of a chair.

Instructions:

1. Tilt your head slowly, nodding forward and backward.

2. Tilt your head slowly from side to side keeping your vision forward, touching your ear to your shoulder.

3. Turn your head to the right, looking over your right shoulder.

4. Return to facing forward, and repeat by turning your head to the left, looking back over your left shoulder.

5. Roll your neck slowly in a circular motion first to the right 2 times, and then back to the left 2 times.

Biceps

To start:

Stand with your feet shoulder width apart. Extend your arms up and out to your sides.

Instructions:

1. Rotate your arms fully from one side then rotate fully to the other side.

Triceps

To start:

Stand with your feet shoulder width apart. Place your arms at your sides.

Instructions:

1. Bring your right arm straight overhead and bend at the elbows, resting on the side of your head.

2. With your other arm grab and pull your elbow. Hold for at least 30 seconds.

3. Repeat on the other side.

Quadriceps (front of thigh) ———————————————

To start:

Stand erect with your feet placed shoulder width apart, facing a wall.

Instructions:

1. Bend your right foot behind your leg toward your glutes.

2. Hold your right foot near the ankle with your left hand, keeping the knee at a comfortable angle.

3. Slowly pull your heel up; you can place your right hand against the wall for support.

4. Pull to the point where you feel the stretch, and hold the position for at least 30 seconds.

5. Change to the other side and repeat.

Hamstrings (back of thigh) ———————————————

To start:

Stand erect with your feet placed shoulder width apart.

Instructions:

1. Bend at the waist, keeping your knees slightly bent, allowing your hands to drop in front of you.

2. Bend to the point where you feel the stretch.

3. Hold the position for at least 30 seconds.

Hips and Glutes: Squat Stretch ———————————

To start:

Stand erect with your feet placed shoulder width apart. Your feet should be point forward.

Instructions:

1. Slowly bend your knees as you squat toward the floor, keeping your feet flat. Keep your knees outside your shoulders and positioned above your toes. Your hands can rest on the floor between your feet.

2. Press with your hips to the point where you feel the stretch, and hold the position for at least 30 seconds.

3. When you come out of the squat, raise your body with your quadriceps and keep a straight back.

Lower back: Fetal Position Stretch

To start:

Lie on your right side with your knees drawn to your chest, head resting on your hands.

Instructions:

1. Use your left arm to pull your left leg higher into the chest.

2. Pull to the point where you feel the stretch in your lower back, and hold the position for at least 30 seconds.

3. Turn over to the other side and repeat.

Calves

To start:

Stand facing a wall.

Instructions:

1. Place your hands on the wall hip-distance apart.

2. Bring one leg forward and bend at the knees.

3. Extend the other leg behind you, and align it with the forward leg. Lean on the forward leg. You should feel a stretch in back of your calf. Hold for at least 30 seconds

4. Repeat on the other side.

COOL-DOWN STRETCHES FOR THE THREE-MONTHS PROGRAM

Wall Stretch

Benefits:

This stretch opens your chest.

To start:

Stand alongside a wall.

Instructions:

1. Hold your arm on the wall and rotate your hand externally.

2. Hold for 30 seconds.

3. Repeat on the other side.

Head Lean

Benefits:

This stretch releases your shoulders.

To start:

Sit up straight on the edge of a chair or a physioball.

Instructions:

1. Lean your head to one side and then the other.

2. Hold for 30 seconds on each side.

Jaw Tuck

Benefits:

This stretches the muscles under the skull at the back of the neck.

To start:

Stand comfortably.

Instructions:

1. Hold your head straight up. Retract the jaw so that it tilts the face slightly forward.

2. Hold for 30 seconds and breathe deeply.

Back Reach

Benefits:

This stretch opens your back.

To start:

Kneel on the floor and place a physioball or exercise bench in front of you.

Instructions:

1. Place one hand on the ball or bench with your arm fully extended. Rotate your hand externally. You should feel a stretch in your back.

2. Hold for 30 seconds.

3. Repeat on the other side.

Wrist Stretch

Benefits:

This stretches your forearms and wrist.

To start:

Stand comfortably with feet shoulder width apart. Extend your arms up and in front of you, palms facing up.

Instructions:

1. Hold your fingertips of the right hand with the left hand.

2. Press the palm of the right hand downward and straighten the elbow.

3. Hold comfortably for 30 seconds, and breathe deeply.

4. Repeat, changing hands.

Bent Knee Lunge

Benefits:

This stretch opens your quadriceps.

To start:

Kneel down with one knee on the floor while the other is flexed at a 90-degree angle.

Instructions:

1. Lunge forward.

2. Hold the position for 30 seconds.

3. Repeat on the other side.

Hamstring Stretch

Benefits:

This exercise stretches your hamstrings.

To start:

Lie on your back with one leg flat on the floor, the other at a 90-degree angle.

Instructions:

1. Raise your bent leg and grab your lower thigh near your knee joint. Straighten out your leg completely.

2. Gently pull your leg toward you to the point where you feel the stretch.

3. Hold the position 30 seconds.

4. Repeat with the other leg.

Note: Use a yoga strap or a belt for a deeper stretch.

Lateral Stride

Benefits:

This exercise stretches your inner thighs.

To start:

Stand erect with your feet wider than shoulder width apart.

Instructions:

1. Place hands on your hips and lean to one side, bending one knee and placing pressure on your hip with your hand.

2. Hold the position for 30 seconds.

3. Repeat with the other leg.

Spine Rotation

Benefits:

This stretch opens your lower back.

To start:

Lie on your back on top of an exercise mat.

Instructions:

1. Rotate one knee over the opposite thigh.

2. Use the hand of your opposite arm to pull your leg gently toward the floor.

3. Extend your other arm out to your side.

4. Pull until you feel the stretch in your lower back.

5. Hold the position for 30 seconds.

6. Turn over to the other side and repeat.

Wall Stretch

Benefits:

This exercise stretches your calves.

To start:

Stand erect facing a wall.

Instructions:

1. Place your hands on the wall hip-distance apart.

2. Bring one leg forward and place the balls of your feet on the wall and lean forward. Keep your legs straight.

3. Extend the other leg behind you. You should feel a stretch in your front calf.

4. Hold the position for 30 seconds.

5. Switch legs and repeat.

COOL DOWN STRETCHES FOR THE ONE-MONTH PROGRAM

Shoulder Blade Squeeze

Benefits:

This stretches your pectoral muscles.

To start:

Stand comfortably with feet shoulder width apart.

Instructions:

Place your hands behind your back and interlock your hands.

Squeeze the shoulder blades together and hold for 30 seconds.

Note: If your hands are below the waist, you will stretch the middle and upper region of your chest.

If your hands are closer to your upper back you will stretch the lower region of your chest.

Rotator Cuff Stretch

Benefits:

This stretches your rotator cuff, the back part of your shoulders muscles.

To start:

Stand comfortably with feet shoulder width apart.

Instructions:

1. Bend the right arm at the elbow and place your left wrist on top of your right elbow.

2. Use the left hand to hold the right elbow, pulling it gently forward.

3. Hold for 30 seconds, breathing deeply.

4. Repeat on the other side.

Note: For a greater stretch, twist the torso to the left.

Sitting Twist

Benefits:

This stretches the spinal rotator muscles, the lower back, and glutes.

To start:

Sit on the floor with the right leg crossed over the left. Use the left elbow to apply very gentle leverage against the right knee. Rest the right hand on the floor for support.

Instructions:

1. Hold for 30 seconds, breathing deeply.

2. Repeat on the other side.

External Rotation Stretch

Benefits:

This stretch works your biceps.

To start:

Stand comfortably with feet shoulder width apart, knees slightly bent, and shoulders back.

Instructions:

1. Hold the arms straight with palms facing toward each other. Turn the elbows outward and rotate the shoulders forward and inward.

2. Hold comfortably for 30 seconds. Breathe deeply.

Ankle Reach

Benefits:

This exercise stretches your hamstrings.

To start:

Sit on the floor with your legs spread apart. Keep your back straight, head up, and knees slightly bent.

Instructions:

1. Lean straight forward over your right leg. Do not round your back.

2. Hold for 30 seconds, and breathe deeply.

3. Repeat on the other side.

Cat Stretch/Back Arch

Benefits:

This stretches your lower back.

To start:

Place your hands and knees on an exercise mat. Keep your feet together.

Instructions:

1. Press the center of your back upward toward the ceiling, like a cat stretching.

2. Hold for 30 seconds, and breathe deeply.

3. Follow immediately with the Back Arch.

Back Arch

Benefits:

This stretches your lower back.

To start:

Press your abdomen toward the floor and arch your lower back

Instructions:

Remain in position from Step #2 of the Cat Stretch.

1. Hold comfortably for 30 seconds, and breathe deeply.

2. Repeat this series 5 times.

Half-Kneeling Shin Stretch

Benefits:

This stretches your shins.

To start:

Kneel on the floor so that your legs are bent at a 90-degree angle.

Instructions:

1. Lay your ankles flat on the floor. Keep your feet together. Do not sit back as it will strain your knees.

2. Hold for 30 seconds.

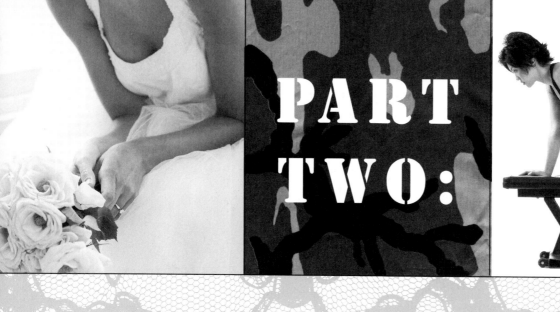

PART TWO:

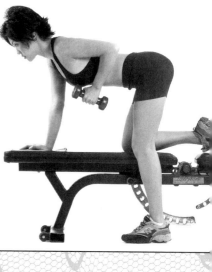

Bootcamp

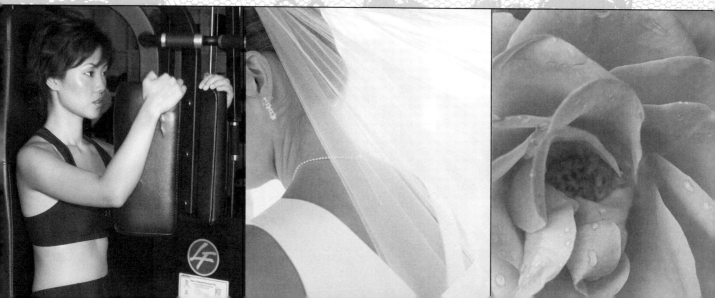

CHAPTER FIVE:

Six Months to the Wedding

Hopefully, your engagement jitters subsided once you stopped drinking coffee. Have you booked the reception hall? Hired the band? Ordered the dress? Don't worry about the size: a good seamstress can always take it in. Now, let's get with the program!

If you are starting this program six months before your wedding day, I want you to focus on three goals:

1. Four days each week, complete the hour-long, integrated workouts in the second half of this chapter. They were designed to get you in great shape quickly.

2. Reduce your food intake so you are getting 500 calories less than you would need to maintain your weight at current levels. (More on that later.)

3. Keep your daily food diary and measurement journal up to date. I want you to enter the following in your measurement journal:

• Your weight, every week

• Your body fat, measured by the skinfold caliper, every other week

• Your girth measurements, every month

Speaking of your vital statistics, keep in mind that a tighter body is not necessarily a lighter body. Muscle mass adds weight. So don't panic if you are only losing a pound a week, even though you are following the diet correctly and working out more than ever before. Your measurements will tell the real story. If the numbers on your scale show little movement, check your measurements weekly, if you have to, to stay motivated. And just be patient—the scale will show a change before long.

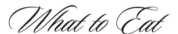

What to Eat

Once you determine your new caloric intake you will remain at that calorie level for the next three months. In Chapter 2, we used the following equation to determine Carol's daily caloric maintenance level: current weight x 14.25 = your daily caloric maintenance level

For example, Carol weighs 160 pounds, her goal is to weigh 130 pounds for her wedding.

160 x 14.25 = 2280

Carol's daily caloric maintenance level is 2280 calories, therefore her reduction in calories would be as follows: 2280 - 20% = 1824 calories per day or 1800 rounded-out.

If you begin to lose more than 2 pounds of body fat a week, you're likely to be losing muscle tissue. Monitor your body fat closely. That is why it is important to measure your body fat every two weeks, to ensure that the weight that is coming off is fat and not muscle tissue. If your body fat test reveals that you are losing muscle, then you need to add some calories back to your diet. You should add back 25 calories per day, for five days, until you reach a 125 calories surplus. For example, if Carol determined that she was losing too much weight too fast, and most of it was lean muscle mass, then she would increase her daily caloric intake to 1949. If you have a slow metabolism, then you will have to make additional adjustments to your daily caloric intake.

Start off by determining how many calories you eat on an average day. Use the following meal plans as a guide to see the caloric content of foods. You might need to find a calorie counting book, like Corrine T. Netzer's *The Complete Book of Food Counts*, so you can see how what you are eating adds up.

Start eating foods featured in the *Bridal Bootcamp*™ Four Food Groups. After five days, you'll be used to eating a bit less, and probably, a bit better. Then you'll be ready to use the meal plan. Each day on the seven-day meal plan is roughly 1800 calories. Refer back to your weight loss caloric intake number in your journal. If your number is less or more than 1800 calories, you will need to modify the meal plans. You can remove or add some foods from your daily five-meal plan throughout the day until you reach your number, but don't skip any of the meals entirely.

For the first week, follow the meal plans exactly. Afterward, you can create your own 1800 calorie days from the sample meals. Here is the way to convert caloric ratios to grams of food. For example Carol determined that she needs to eat 1800 calories per day to start losing body fat. And the nutrient ratio is roughly 50/30/20. Remember:

1 gram of carbohydrates = 4 calories

1 gram of protein = 4 calories

1 gram of fat = 9 calories

Nutrient Ratio Calculator

Carbohydrate (1800) x (.50) = 900 grams

Protein (1800) x (.30) = 540 grams

Fat (1800) x (.20) = 360 grams

Therefore, Carol should have the following:

Carbohydrate - 900 calories ÷ 4 cal/gr = 225 gr

Protein - 540 calories ÷ 4 cal/gr = 135 gr

Fat - 360 calories ÷ 9 cal/gr = 40 gr

We all know that this is not a perfect world. Therefore, I'll allow you one cheat meal per week after you have lost 5 pounds of fat. Try to make it a Sunday, so that you are back on schedule by Monday. Don't let your cheat meal turn into a cheat day!

SEVEN DAY WEDDING MEAL PLAN

Everyday morning start your day with the Water Method listed in Chapter 2. Wait at least thirty minutes, then eat breakfast. Remember to keep a daily food diary. It is extremely important to monitor your daily caloric intake. Also keep in mind that these calorie counts are for "cooked" foods. The brown rice, for example, refers to a cup of cooked brown rice, rather than the uncooked, which would expand to much more than one cup when cooked.

Day 1

Meal 1 (cereal and milk)	Protein	Carbohydrates	Fat	Calories
1½ cup low calorie breakfast cereal	7.35	28.05	.15	147
1 cup 2% low fat milk	8.13	11.7	4.68	121
1 multivitamin				
1 calcium/mag				
Total calories				268
Total calories %	23	59	16	
Meal 2 (yogurt and fruit)	Protein	Carbohydrates	Fat	Calories
1 cup of strawberries	.88	10.2	.53	49
6 oz. low fat yogurt	9.0	12.75	3.0	112
Total calories				161
Total calories %	24	56	19	

Meal 3 (tuna pocket)	Protein	Carbohydrates	Fat	Calories
1 whole wheat pita bread	4.4	24.8	1.16	120
3 oz. tuna fish in water	22.7	0	2.09	116
1 tbs. low calorie mayonnaise	.05	2.5	3.0	36
1 apple	.4	32.2	.76	137
1 multivitamin				
1 calcium				
Total calories				409
Total calories %	26	58	15	

Meal 4 (Peanut Butter Paradise Smoothie)	Protein	Carbohydrates	Fat	Calories
8 oz. vanilla soymilk	7.0	18.0	5.	150
½ tbs. peanut butter	2.25	1.5	4	47
1 banana	1.17	26.8	.55	116
1 scoop Gotein protein	12	2.0	0	55
Total calories				369
Total calories %	24	52	23	

Meal 5 (chicken and brown rice with veggies)	Protein	Carbohydrates	Fat	Calories
1½ cup long grain brown rice	7.56	67.5	2.64	324
4 oz. grilled chicken breast	34.32	0	3.95	180
1 cup broccoli	4.65	7.89	55	43
2 tbs. low calorie Italian dressing	0	2	4	44
1 antioxidant				
Total calories				592
Total calories %	31	52	16	
Grand total calories				1800

Day 2

Meal 1 (egg and whole grain toast)	Protein	Carbohydrates	Fat	Calories
3 egg whites	12.3	1.21	0	54
1 whole egg	6.25	.61	5	72
2 slices whole wheat bread	5.16	26.8	2.32	147
1 tbs. jelly	0	12	0	48
1 multivitamin				
1 cal/mag				
Total calories				322
Total calories %	29	50	20	

Meal 2 (Strawberry Fields Smoothie)	Protein	Carbohydrates	Fat	Calories
8 oz. apple juice	.15	.29	.27	116
1 cup strawberries	.88	10.2	.53	49
¼ cup low fat vanilla yogurt	6.03	8.54	2.01	75
½ banana	.59	13.4	.27	58
2 tsp. flaxseed oil	0	0	9.08	80
1 scoop Gotein protein	12.0	2.0	0	55
Total calories				434
Total calories %	18	58	25	

Meal 3 (turkey sandwich)	Protein	Carbohydrates	Fat	Calories
3 oz. fresh turkey breast	16.05	.32	4.34	104
2 slices whole grain bread	5.16	26.8	2.32	147
1 tbs. mustard	.13	1.16	2.31	24
1 orange	1.23	15.5	.16	68
1 multivitamin				
1 cal/mag				
Total calories				345
Total calories %	26	50	23	
Meal 4 (chicken burrito)	Protein	Carbohydrates	Fat	Calories
1 corn tortilla	1.71	14	.75	66
1 cup brown rice	2.52	22.5	.88	108
2 oz. chicken breast	18.48	0	2.13	97
Total calories				271
Total calories %	33	53	12	

Meal 5 (pasta with turkey meatballs)	Protein	Carbohydrates	Fat	Calories
1 cup spinach	5.35	6.75	0	48
2 oz. tomato sauce marinara	.76	4.08	.1	20
1 cup pasta cooked	8.35	49.75	1.17	246
3 oz. ground turkey	17.6	0	.8	80
1 tsp. olive oil	0	0	4.7	43
1 antioxidant				
Total calories				437
Total calories %	29	55	13	
Grand total calories				1811

Meal 1 (strawberry granola fruit parfait)	Protein	Carbohydrates	Fat	Calories
½ cup blueberries	.49	10.2	.28	40
½ cup strawberries	.44	5.1	.27	24
3 oz. low fat granola	2.9	19.1	4.9	126
6 oz. plain low fat yogurt	13.5	19.13	4.5	168
1 multivitamin				
1 cal/mag				
Total calories				359
Total calories %	19	59	24	
Meal 2 (Brazilian Rain smoothie)	Protein	Carbohydrates	Fat	Calories
½ cup orange juice	.87	12.9	.25	55
½ cup pineapple juice	.4	17.3	.1	70
½ mango diced (fresh or frozen)	.53	17.6	.28	75
2 scoops Gotein protein	24	4	0	110
Total calories				390
Total calories %	26	53	22	

Meal 3 (chicken & broccoli)	Protein	Carbohydrates	Fat	Calories
1 cup broccoli	4.65	7.89	.55	43
1 tbs. low-cal French dressing	0	2.1	2.5	31
1 cup brown rice	5.04	45	1.76	216
2 oz. grilled chicken breast	18.48	0	2.13	97
1 multivitamin				
1 cal/mag				
Total calories				388
Total calories %	29	56	16	
Meal 4 (protein drink)	Protein	Carbohydrates	Fat	Calories
8 oz. vanilla soy milk	7	18	5.0	150
1 banana	1.17	26.8	.55	116
1 scoop Gotein protein	12	2	0	55
Total calories				321
Total calories %	25	58	12	

Meal 5 (turkey meatloaf and brown rice)	Protein	Carbohydrates	Fat	Calories
1 cup broccoli	4.65	7.89	.55	43
1 cup brown rice	5.04	45	1.76	216
2 oz. turkey meat loaf	11.0	0	.5	50
1 tsp butter	.04	0	3.83	34
1 antioxidant				
Total calories				344
Total calories %	24	61	17	
Grand total calories				1804

Day 4

Meal 1 (whole grain cereal with soy milk)	Protein	Carbohydrates	Fat	Calories
1 cup whole grain cereal	4.79	21.98	2.03	124
1 cup vanilla soy milk	7	18	5	150
1 multivitamin				
1 cal/mag				
Total calories				274
Total calories %	17	58	23	

Meal 2 (rice cakes and peanut butter)	Protein	Carbohydrates	Fat	Calories
3 rice cakes (any flavor)	4.2	43.8	1.8	210
1 tbs. peanut butter	4.5	3	8	95
1 scoop Gotein protein mixed w/ 8oz. of water	12.0	2	0	55
Total calories				360
Total calories %	23	54	24	
Meal 3 (tuna sandwich on whole wheat bread)	Protein	Carbohydrates	Fat	Calories
2 slices of whole wheat bread	5.16	26.8	2.32	147
3 oz. tuna fish in water	22.7	0	2.09	116
1 tbs. low fat mayonnaise	.05	2.5	3	36
1 orange	1.23	15.5	.16	68
1 multivitamin				
1 cal/mag				
Total calories				367
Total calories %	31	48	18	

Meal 4 (Cleanser Smoothie)	Protein	Carbohydrates	Fat	Calories
4 oz. cranberry juice	0	18.2	.13	72
4 oz. water	0	0	0	0
½ banana	.59	13.4	.27	58
½ cup blueberries	.49	10.2	.28	40
½ cup strawberries	.44	5.1	.27	24
¼ cup low fat vanilla yogurt	2.7	3.83	.9	33
1 tsp. flaxseed oil	0	0	4.54	40
2 scoops Gotein protein	24	4	0	110
Total calories				379
Total calories %	29	57	15	
Meal 5 (turkey and roasted peppers wrap)	Protein	Carbohydrates	Fat	Calories
1 corn tortilla	1.71	14	.75	66
4 oz. ground turkey	22	0	1.0	100
2 oz. roasted peppers	1	7.6	.2	32
3 tbs. onion	1.23	9.15	0	40
1 tsp. olive oil	0	0	4.7	43
1 apple	.4	32.2	.76	137
1 antioxidant				

Meal 5 (continued)	Protein	Carbohydrates	Fat	Calories
Total calories				419
Total calories %	25	55	20	
Grand total calories				1800

Day 5

Meal 1 (bagel and eggs)	Protein	Carbohydrates	Fat	Calories
1 whole wheat bagel (scooped out)	5.88	30.4	.82	143
2 tbs. low fat cream cheese	3.18	2.1	5.28	69
3 egg whites	9.84	.96	0	43
1 multivitamin				
1 cal/mag				
Total calories				255
Total calories %	29	52	21	

Meal 2 (Berry Blend)	Protein	Carbohydrates	Fat	Calories
12 oz. vanilla soy milk	10.5	27	7.5	225
1/2 cup blueberries	.49	10.2	.28	40
1/2 cup raspberries	.56	7.05	.34	33
1 tbs. honey	.03	8.7	0	32
1 scoop Gotein protein	12	2	0	55
Total calories				386
Total calories %	24	56	18	

Meal 3 (chicken salad with seven grain bread)	Protein	Carbohydrates	Fat	Calories
2 slices whole grain bread	5.16	26.8	2.32	147
2 oz. shredded chicken	18.48	0	2.13	97
1 tbs. low cal. mayonnaise	.05	2.5	3	36
1 multivitamin				
1 cal/mag				
Total calories				371
Total calories %	27	53	19	

Meal 4 (The American Smoothie)	Protein	Carbohydrates	Fat	Calories
12 oz. organic nonfat milk	12.5	17.9	.66	128
1 tbs. peanut butter	4.5	3	8	95
1 banana	1.17	26.8	.55	116
3 tbs. oatmeal or rolled oats	2.5	9	1	50
1 scoop Gotein protein	12	2	0	55
Total calories				444
Total calories %	29	52	20	
Meal 5 (pasta and shrimp)	Protein	Carbohydrates	Fat	Calories
1 cup spinach	5.35	6.75	0	48
1 cup pasta cooked any kind	6.68	39.8	.94	197
2 oz. shrimp	11.5	.85	1	56
1 tsp olive oil	0	0	4.7	43
1 antioxidant				
Total calories				345
Total calories %	27	54	19	
Grand total calories				1803

Meal 1 (oatmeal and egg whites)	Protein	Carbohydrates	Fat	Calories
1 tbs. maple syrup	0	13.4	.04	52
1 cup oatmeal cooked	6.38	26.57	2.46	152
3 egg whites	9.84	.96	0	43
1 tsp butter	.04	0	3.83	34
1 multivitamin				
1 calcium/mag				
Total calories				282
Total calories %	23	57	20	
Meal 2 (Java Junkies Smoothie)	Protein	Carbohydrates	Fat	Calories
8 oz. vanilla soy milk	7	18	5	150
½ banana	.59	13.40	.27	58
1 tbs. peanut butter	4.5	3	8	95
1 scoop instant coffee	0	0	0	0
1 tbs. honey	.06	17.4	0	64
1 scoop Gotein protein	12	2	0	55
Total calories				422
Total calories %	22	50	28	

Meal 3 (chicken tortilla)	Protein	Carbohydrates	Fat	Calories
1 tortilla 8-inch	3.08	19.7	2.51	115
2 oz. chicken breast	18.48	0	2.13	97
1 tsp. olive oil	0	0	4.7	43
1 apple	.4	32.2	.76	137
1 multivitamin				
1 cal/mag				
Total calories				392
Total calories %	22	52	23	
Meal 4 (protein drink)	Protein	Carbohydrates	Fat	Calories
8 oz. vanilla soy milk	7	18	5	150
6 frozen strawberries	1.32	15.3	.8	73
1 scoop Gotein protein	12	2	0	55
Total calories				278
Total calories %	29	50	18	

Meal 5 (steak and potatoes)	Protein	Carbohydrates	Fat	Calories
1 cup of cauliflower	3.45	7.65	.84	42
1 medium potato baked with skin	4.64	51	.2	220
3 oz. beef sirloin	25.8	0	6.81	171
1 antioxidant				
Total calories				433
Total calories %	31	54	16	
Grand total calories				1810

Day 7

Meal 1 (French toast)	Protein	Carbohydrates	Fat	Calories
2 slices of bread	5.16	26.8	2.32	147
½ cup egg beaters	10	2	0	50
1 tsp butter	.04	0	3.83	34
1 tbs. maple syrup	0	13.4	.04	52
1 multivitamin				
1 cal/mag				
Total calories				284
Total calories %	21	59	19	

Meal 2 (rice cake w tuna)	Protein	Carbohydrates	Fat	Calories
3 rice cakes	2.1	21.9	.9	105
3 oz. tuna fish in water	22.7	0	2.09	116
1 tbs. mayo	.05	2.5	3	36
1 cup apple sauce	.42	27.6	.12	104
Total calories				361
Total calories %	27	57	15	
Meal 3 (veal and veggies)	Protein	Carbohydrates	Fat	Calories
1 cup brown rice	5.04	45	1.765	216
½ cup mixed veggies	3.24	14.82	.17	66
2 oz. veal	20.5	0	3.6	119
1 tsp. olive oil	0	0	4.7	43
1 multivitamin				
1 cal/mag				
Total calories				445
Total calories %	25	53	20	

Meal 4 (protein drink)	Protein	Carbohydrates	Fat	Calories
8 oz. apple juice	.15	29	.27	116
½ banana	.59	13.4	.27	58
1 tsp. flaxseed oil	0	0	4.54	40
1 scoop Gotein protein	24	4	0	110
Total calories				324
Total calories %	30	57	14	
Meal 5 (Salmon and yams)	Protein	Carbohydrates	Fat	Calories
1 cup zucchini	1.15	7.07	.09	28
1 cup yams	3.44	48.6	.22	206
3 oz. Atlantic salmon	21.6	0	6.9	154
1 antioxidant				
Total calories				389
Total calories %	26	57	16	
Grand total calories				1804

The Wedding Workout at Six Months

If it has been a while since you exercised vigorously, I strongly suggest that you approach this program with gentleness in mind. Don't push yourself too hard the first week or so. Get used to the idea of a regular exercise routine, then gradually increase the difficulty as the weeks go on. No pain, no gain is not part of *Bridal Bootcamp*™.

The six-month workout should be done three times a week, with an additional day of cardiovascular, abdominal work, and stretching. The perfect routine in seven days would be two days on, one day off, two days on, two days off. The routines are designed to take an hour. Assume that you will need at least another thirty minutes the first week or so, as you learn the exercises.

Important: Keep your rest time in between sets 30 seconds.

Day 1: 1 hour

Day 2: 1 hour

Day 3: Rest

Day 4: 1 hour

Day 5: 35 minutes (Aerobic training, abdominal work, and stretching)

Day 6: Rest

Day 7: Rest

Determining Your Heart Rate

Before you begin exercising, you need to determine what your target heart rate should be. To work out at level that is both safe and effective, I recommend using target heart rate training. To determine your heart rate, I use the Karvonen formula.

1. The first step is to determine your resting heart rate. This can be done first thing in the morning. Place your index and middle fingers lightly on your carotid artery, which is found on the neck just below your jaw, or on top of your wrist with palms facing upward. Wait until you feel a pulse. Count the beats for

10 seconds and multiply that number by 6. That will determine your resting heart rate. For example, if you count 12 beats in 10 seconds, 12 x 6 = 72 beats per minute.

2. Next, determine your maximum heart rate (MHR). The MHR is determined by subtracting one's age from 220. For example, Lori, a thirty-five-year-old woman, subtracts 35 from 220.

    220 - 35 = 185

3. Next, subtract the resting rate from the MHR.

    Resting heart rate =72

    Maximum heart rate = 185

    185 - 72 = 113

You need to train between 60 and 85 percent of your maximum heart rate. To arrive at these numbers, multiply the result (113) by the desired intensity level.

    For example, 113 x 60% = 67.8 and 113 x 85% = 96.05

4. Finally add, the resting heart rate to this result. For example, 72 + 96.05= 168 (rounding off). That means that Lori should be training between 140 - 168 beats per minute, which is more than double her resting heartrate. At this rate she will be in her fat burning zone.

USING THE HEART RATE MONITOR

Your heart rate monitor is a necessary piece of equipment during the Bridal Bootcamp™ Workouts. Purchase a heart rate monitor that also determines your heart rate as a percentage of your maximum heart rate. To use, first moisten the back of the monitor. Before you get dressed, strap the monitor underneath your chest. If you can slide a finger between the strap and your body, the monitor is too loose. Put on the wrist monitor and face it toward the chest piece. This will activate the monitor and in a few seconds your heart rate will appear on the wristband. Check your wristband at several points throughout the workouts in order to increase or decrease intensity as needed.

The Gym Workout

Daily Warm-Ups

Heart rate: 60% of maximum heart rate

Duration: 5 minutes

Choose from the following activities for a five-minute warm-up routine:

- Treadmill
- Recumbent bicycle
- Stair climber
- Elliptical climber

Dynamic Stretch

Heart rate: 60 % of maximum heart rate

Duration: 5 minutes

Warm-Ups

- Flutter Kick, page 47
- Mountain Climbers, page 47
- Walking Lunge with Twist, page 48
- Squat Thrusts, page 48
- Jumping Jacks, page 49

Progress from one exercise to the next without resting in between. Then move to the abdominal drills.

Abdominal Drills

Heart Rate: 55% of maximum heart rate

Duration: 5 minutes

Warm up by stretching over a physioball, or doing a Cobra Posture stretch, page 56. Then choose a different abdominal group set for each day of the four days of your workout.

Abdominal Group 1

- Reverse Crunch: 3 sets, 15 repetitions each, page 84
- Cross Body Crunch: 3 sets, 15 repetitions each, page 58
- Basic Crunch: 3 sets, 15 repetitions each, page 59

Abdominal Group 2

- Vertical-Bench Leg Raise: 3 sets, 15 repetitions each, page 79
- Oblique Crunch: 3 sets, 15 repetitions each, page 60
- V-Ups: 3 sets, 15 repetitions each, page 65

Abdominal Group 3

- Scissors Kick: 2 sets, 20 repetitions each, page 66

- Double Crunch: 2 sets, 20 repetitions each, page 61
- Side Bend: 2 sets, 15 repetitions each, page 67
- Cross Over Split Leg Crunch: 2 sets, 20 repetitions each, page 62
- Hands Over Head Crunch: 2 sets, 20 repetitions each, page 71

Abdominal Group 4

These exercises are a bit more difficult. If you are a novice or do not have the abdominal strength yet, rotate routines 1 through 3 until you are able to do routine 4. Do this routine on Day 5 of your weekly workouts. Start with the aerobic routine, then Abdominal Group 4, and finish with the post workout stretch.

- Reverse Crunch on Incline Board: 2 sets, 15 repetitions each, page 84
- Reverse Crunch with Physioball: 2 sets, 20 repetitions each, page 68
- Decline-Bench Twisting Crunch: 2 sets, 15 repetitions each, page 78
- Hip Thrust: 2 sets, 15 repetitions each, page 74
- Cable Crunch with Rope: 2 sets, 15 repetitions each, page 81

Strength Training

Heart Rate: 65% of your maximum heart rate
Duration: 20 minutes

The strength training system for the six month workout consists of three total body workouts per week. Each workout emphasizes the same body part in a slightly different way. I have listed three workouts. For the fourth day, you will do your aerobic training, ab work, and stretching routine only.

Strength Training Group 1

- Leg Press: 2 sets, 20 repetitions, page 89
- Lying Leg Curl: 2 sets, 15 repetitions, page 92
- Barbell Squats: 2 sets, 10 repetitions, page 112
- Seated Cable Rows: 2 sets, 20 repetitions, page 97
- Upright Rows: 2 sets, 12 repetitions each, page 144
- Overhead Lateral Raise: 2 sets, 15 repetitions, page 143
- Flat Dumbbell Flyes: 2 sets, 15 repetitions, page 125
- Triceps Pressdown: 3 sets, 12 repetitions, page 98
- Dumbbell Concentration Curls: 2 sets, 15 repetitions, page 126
- Seated Calf Raise: 2 sets, 20 repetitions, page 94

Strength Training Group 2

- Smith Machine Squats: 2 sets 20 repetitions, page 103
- Leg Extensions: 2 sets, 15 repetitions each, page 105
- One Arm Dumbbell Rows: 2 sets, 15 repetitions each, page 127
- Incline Dumbbell Press: 2 sets, first set 15, then 12 repetitions each, page 128
- Pec Dec: 2 sets, 15 repetitions each, page 106
- Front Dumbbell Raise: 2 sets, 15 repetitions, page 138
- Seated Dumbbell Press: 2 sets, 12 repetitions, page 129
- One Arm Reverse-Grip Pressdown: 3 sets, 15 repetitions, page 99
- One Arm Preacher Dumbbell Curls: 2 sets, 15 repetitions each, page 123
- Leg Press Calf Raise: 2 sets, 20 repetitions each, page 93

Strength Training Group 3

- Hack Squat: 2 sets, 20 repetitions, page 108
- Barbell Lunges: 2 sets, 15 repetitions each, page 109
- Stiff-Leg Deadlift: 2 sets, 10 repetitions, page 133
- Flat Dumbbell Press: 2 sets, 15 repetitions, page 110
- Wide Grip Front Pulldown: 2 sets, 10 repetitions each, page 117
- Bent-Over Lateral Raise: 2 sets, 12 repetitions, page 131
- Shoulder Press Machine: 2 sets, 12 repetitions, page 116
- Bench Dip: 2 sets, 12 repetitions each, page 90
- Standing Barbell Curls: 2 sets, 12 repetitions each, page 111
- Standing Calf Raise: 2 sets, 20 repetitions, page 96

Aerobic Workout:
High-intensity Interval Training

Heart rate: 70–75% of maximum heart rate

Duration: 20 minutes

For the six-month program, choose one machine and stick with it for the month. The following month choose another, and finally a third machine. (This program lasts three months, bringing you to the three-month workout.) If you go back to a machine you've previously done, be sure to allow yourself at least two months in between.

High-intensity Interval Training

High-intensity interval training is the most efficient form of cardiovascular work. The workout is composed of a warm-up, intervals, and cooldown. The interval section is composed of an exertion scale rating from 1 to 10: 1 representing little exertion and 10 an all out effort. The level of exertion refers to the intensity of your workout, and will depend on your level of fitness. Start with a level you feel comfortable with, and increase your intensity as you become more fit.

You will never do more than twenty minutes of this type of exercise a day. When you work at high intensity, you can burn a maximum amount of calories in a minimum amount of time. Also, extended aerobic activity produces cortisol, which is a catabolic agent that breaks muscle protein, causing the burning of muscle tissue.

A true cardiovascular workout is considered to be an aerobic activity, which increases your oxygen intake and therefore increases your heart rate. Aerobic activity that is sustained at a higher percentage of your maximum heart rate (65 to 85 percent) will burn more calories more efficiently. Cardiovascular exercise burns calories and body fat in a different way than strength training. It utilizes body fat and carbohydrates for energy, creating a significant amount of energy for long periods of time.

If you haven't exercised recently, try working within 60 to 65 percent of your maximum heart rate. Once you adapt to the exercise intensity level, increase your workout intensity. By changing the intensity every week, you will avoid plateaus and continue to lose body fat.

Treadmill

Program: Random (Choose this program so the machine randomly changes the incline level)

Incline: 4

Important: Monitor your heart rate to the levels recommended in the chart below. If you see that it is going up too high, lower your exertion level by one unit at a time.

Duration in minutes	Description	Target Heart Rate	Speed
1	warm-up	60%	3.5
2	low intensity	65%	4.0
2	medium intensity	65%	4.2
2	high intensity	70%	4.4
2	high intensity	70%	4.6
1	recovery	60%	3.5
2	low intensity	65%	4.0
2	medium intensity	65%	4.2
2	high intensity	70%	4.4
2	high intensity	70%	4.6
2	cool-down	60%	3.5

After your initial one minute warm-up, begin increasing the intensity by 2 levels every two minutes, until your reach the recovery stage where you decrease the intensity level. Stick with the same level of intensity for at least one week. After that, begin to increase your intensity level by 2 units each week.

For other types of equipment, start with a level that you are able to do based on your endurance. Then, increase the level by 1. Only the treadmill can increase the speed by half points. The stair climber, bike and elliptical machine can have their intensity increased by 1's.

Post Workout Stretching:

Heart rate: 50% of maximum heart rate

Duration: 5 minutes

Note: For post workout purposes, static stretching is recommended. Instead of dynamic stretching, where you moved through total joint motion, this time you will hold a position for at least 30 seconds.

- Chest, see page 155
- Shoulders, see page 155
- Back: Folded Leaf Posture, see page 155
- Neck, see page 156
- Biceps, see page 156
- Triceps, see page 156
- Quadriceps (front of thigh), see page 157
- Hamstrings (back of thigh), see page 157
- Hips and Glutes: Squat Stretch, see page 157
- Lower back: Fetal Position Stretch, see page 158
- Calves, see page 158

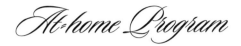

At-home Program

The home program is similar to the gym program, with changes made to adjust for the lack of professional equipment.

Daily Warm-Ups

Heart Rate: 60% of maximum heart rate

Duration: 5 minutes

Jog in place while you hold your arms out to your sides. Then try to rotate your arms clockwise as you jog. Jog for two minutes. Then proceed immediately to jumping jacks, without resting, and continue for another three minutes.

Dynamic Stretch

Heart rate: 60 % of maximum heart rate

Duration: 5 minutes

Warm-Ups

- Flutter Kick, page 47
- Mountain Climbers, page 47
- Walking Lunge with Squat Twist, page 48
- Squat Thrusts, page 48
- Jumping Jacks, page 49

Progress from one exercise to the next without resting in between. Be sure to stretch.

Repeat the entire circuit twice before moving to the abdominal drills.

Abdominal Drills

Heart Rate: 55% of maximum heart rate

Duration: 5 minutes

Warm up by stretching over a physioball, or doing a Cobra Posture stretch, page 00. Then choose a different abdominal group set for each day of the four days of your workout.

Abdominal Group 1 at Home

- Reverse Crunch: 3 sets, 15 repetitions each, page 75
- Cross Body Crunch: 3 sets, 15 repetitions each, page 58
- Basic Crunch: 3 sets, 15 repetitions each, page 59

Abdominal Group 2 at Home

- Bent Leg Hip-Raise: 3 sets, 15 repetitions each, page 69
- Oblique Crunch: 3 sets, 15 repetitions each, page 60
- V-Ups: 3 sets, 15 repetitions each, page 65

Abdominal Group 3 at Home

- Scissors Kick: 2 sets, 20 repetitions each, page 66

- Double Crunch: 2 sets, 20 repetitions each, page 61

- Side Bend: 2 sets, 15 repetitions each, page 67

- Cross Over Split Leg Crunch: 2 sets, 20 repetitions each, page 62

- Hands Overhead Crunch: 2 sets, 20 repetitions each, page 71

Abdominal Group 4 at Home

- Reverse Crunch with Physioball: 3 sets, 20 repetitions each, page 68

- Side Jackknife: 3 sets, 15 repetitions each, page 76

- Hip Thrust: 3 sets, 15 repetitions each, page 74

- Thigh-Slide Crunch: 3 sets, 15 repetitions each, page 64

Strength Training

Heart rate: 65% of maximum heart rate

Duration: 20 minutes

The strength training system for the six month workout consists of three total body workouts per week. Each workout emphasizes the same body part in a slightly different way. I have listed three workouts. For the fourth day you are to do your aerobic training, ab workout, and stretching routine only.

Note: You will need free weights and a physioball for these routines.

Strength Training Group 1 at Home

- Physioball Dumbbell Squats: 3 sets, 15 repetitions each, page 132

- Dumbbell Lunges: 2 sets, 15 repetitions each, page 142

- Bent Over Dumbbell Rows: 2 sets, 15 repetitions each, page 127

- Upright Rows: 2 sets, 12 repetitions each, page 144

- Side Lateral Dumbbell Raise: 2 sets, 12 repetitions each, page 147

- Flat Dumbbell Flyes: repetitions: 12 repetitions each, page 125

- Physioball One Arm Dumbbell Extensions:

2 sets, 15 repetitions each, page 134

- Physioball Dumbbell Concentration Curls: 2 sets, 15 repetitions each, page 126

Strength Training Group 2 at Home

- Dumbbell Squats: 3 sets, 15 repetitions, page 141

- Alternating Dumbbell Lunges: 3 sets, 15 repetitions, page 142

- Good Mornings: 2 sets, 15 repetitions, page 137

- Physioball Push-Ups, 2 sets, 10 repetitions each, page 150

- Alternating Front Dumbbell Raise: 2 sets, 12 repetitions each, page 145

- Chair Dip, 2 sets, 10 repetitions each, page 139

- Standing Dumbbell Curls: 2 sets, 15 repetitions each, page 140

- Standing One Leg Raise: 2 sets, 20 repetitions, page 135

Strength Training Group 3 at Home

- Walking Dumbbell Lunges: Walk the length of a room twice (back and forth), page 142

- Stiff-Leg Deadlift: 2 sets, 15 repetitions, page 133

- Flat Dumbbell Chest Flyes: 2 sets, 12 repetitions, page 125

- Bent Over Lateral Raise: 2 sets, first 12, then 10 repetitions each, page 131

- Front Dumbbell Raise: 2 sets, 10 repetitions each, page 138

- Standing Dumbbell Kickback: 2 sets, 15 repetitions each, page 146

- Dumbbell Concentration Curls: 2 sets, first 15, then 12 repetitions each, page 126

- Standing One Leg Calf Raise: 2 sets, 20 repetitions each, page 135

Aerobic Workout: High-intensity Interval Training

Heart rate: 70 to 75% of maximum heart rate

Duration: 20 minutes

If you own professional gym equipment like a stair climber or treadmill, then do all twenty minutes on one machine following the instructions from the "At Gym Workout."

If you don't own cardiovascular equipment, use a jump rope. You will get an excellent workout and burn lots of calories. If your endurance level is high, aim to do twenty minutes of interval jump rump training. Start at a slow pace. After a minute of jumping rope, pick up the pace. After two minutes, slow down. This is your recovery time. After a minute of rest, pick up the pace again.

If your endurance level is low, start by doing a maximum of five minutes. Increase your speed and your total minutes weekly.

Another option is to in-line skate, or use a traditional bike for ten minutes, followed by ten minutes of power walking or running. No matter which exercise you choose, you still must monitor your heart rate: strive for a 70 to75 percent of your maximum heart rate.

Post Workout Stretching:

Heart rate: 55% of maximum heart rate

Duration: 5 Minutes

Post Workout Stretching:

Heart rate: 50% of maximum heart rate

Duration:5 minutes

Note: For post workout purposes, static stretching is recommended. Instead of dynamic stretching, where you moved through total joint motion, this time you will hold a position for at least 30 seconds.

- Chest, page 155
- Shoulders, page 155
- Back, Folded Leaf Posture, page 155
- Neck, page 156
- Biceps, see page 156
- Triceps, see page 156
- Quadriceps (front of thigh), page 157
- Hamstrings (back of thigh), page 157
- Hips and Glutes: Squat Stretch, page 157
- Lower back: Fetal Position Stretch, page 158
- Calves, page 158

During the post workout stretch, your body might begin to feel like you've done too much. When you work out hard, your body will get sore, especially during the first few weeks. If you experience muscle stiffness, use a heating pad or, better yet, take a warm shower immediately following your post workout stretching.

You have now completed the first three months of your program. Take five days off and do nothing. Let your body rest. You deserve it!

CHAPTER SIX:

Three Months to the Wedding

Now that you are three months into Bootcamp, you should feel stronger, more agile, and hopefully leaner. Your body has gotten over the initial shock of taking in less calories, and you should be coasting through the week, following the meal plan, and taking your vitamins.

Just when you are getting comfortable, I'm going to shock your system again. The next three months should prove to be a bit more challenging, in both on the diet and exercise program. To begin, take a new set of photographs like you did at the beginning of the program and compare your body then and now.

Take your girth measurements, and compare the totals as well as the individual measurements. If you have been following the program rigorously, you should see specific changes. Your legs and abs are leaner, your glutes are tighter, and your arms are firmer. Most important, your body fat is lower.

Throughout this period, please remember to keep your measurement journal up-to-date, by entering the following:

- Your weight, every week.
- Your body fat, measured by the skinfold caliper, every other week.
- Your girth measurements, every month.

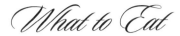

What to Eat

If you've been good, your hard work has paid off. If you've been lax, then you only have yourself to blame. You're getting married in three months. It's now or never. Choose a reward system that works for you, as long as you don't reward your efforts with fatty food. For the next three months, allow yourself only one cheat meal every two weeks.

As you know, carbohydrates are the best energy source. That's why it is important to get the right amount of carbohydrates in every meal. As we discussed earlier, some carbohydrates are better than others. Another change you'll make is to eliminate all high glycemic carbohydrates from your diet. Focus on the low and medium glycemic carbohydrates, especially the ones high in fiber. The following is a list of food grouped by their glycemic index.

Low	Medium	High
Breads		
Sprouted wheat	Rye	French
Pumpernickel	Pita	White
Sourdough	Whole Wheat	Bagel
Fruits		
Apple	Cantaloupe	Watermelon
Berries	Pineapple	Dried dates
Orange	Mango	Banana
Peach	Papaya	
Pear	Plum	
Vegetables		
Kidney beans	Peas	Carrots
Lentils	Baked beans	Corn
Chickpeas	Pinto beans	Potato

We must also begin deducting calories again. First, we must recalculate your daily caloric maintenance level to see what your maximum caloric allotment should be. Then, we will deduct 500 calories from your new caloric maintenance level.

Many women hit a diet plateau. This is because their body is now used to working with less calories. If your daily caloric maintenance level has changed, you'll see right away why you may plateau during the six-month workout.

For example, after doing our calculations in Chapter 2 we determined that Carol's caloric maintenance level was 2280, and reduced her calories by 20 percent to roughly 1800 calories. She began eating 1800 calories at the start of the six-month meal plan when she weighed 160 pounds. Three month later she weighs 145 pounds, and is having a harder time losing body fat. So she needs to reduce her calories by another 20 percent.

Carol's calorie allowance = 1800 calories
1800 ÷ 20% = 1440 (round off to 1500 calories)

Carol should now consume 1500 calories per day.

Each day on the three-month meal plan will be roughly 1500 calories. Refer back to your weight loss caloric intake number in your journal. If your number is not 1500 calories, you will need to modify the meals plans by eating 20 percent less than your daily caloric allowance. You can remove some food items throughout the day until you reach your number, but don't skip any of the meals entirely.

For the first week, follow the meal plans exactly. Afterward, you can create your own 1500 calorie days from the sample meals. Use the guidelines to mix the appropriate four groups to get to the proper ratio of 50 percent carbohydrates, 30 percent protein, 20 percent fat.

If you begin to lose more than 2 pounds of body fat a week, you're likely to be losing muscle tissue. Monitor your body fat closely. If this is occurring, add back 25 calories a day until you reach a 100 surplus calories.

1500 CALORIE SEVEN-DAY MEAL PLAN

Day 1

Meal 1 (oatmeal and egg whites)	Protein	Carbohydrates	Fat	Calories
1 cup of oatmeal cooked	6.38	26.57	2.46	152
3 egg whites	9.84	.96	0	43
1 teaspoon butter	.04	0	3.83	34
1 multivitamin				
1 calcium/mag				
Total calories				230
Total calories %	28	47	24	
Meal 2 (protein drink)	Protein	Carbohydrates	Fat	Calories
1 scoop Gotein protein	25	0	0	100
½ banana	.59	13.4	.27	58
1 teaspoon flaxseed oil	0	0	4.54	40
8 oz. of water				
Total calories				198
Total calories %	51	27	21	

Meal 3 (flounder over barley)	Protein	Carbohydrates	Fat	Calories
2 cups salad, Romaine	2.54	10	.7	49
1 tomato small	1.05	5.71	.41	25
½ cup of barley	2.56	19.3	.41	96
3 oz. flounder	19.11	0	1.21	87
1 tablespoon dressing oil and vinegar	0	1.7	3	34
1 multivitamin				
1 calcium/mag				
Total calories				293
Total calories %	34	50	19	
Meal 4 (protein drink)	Protein	Carbohydrates	Fat	Calories
1 scoop Gotein protein	25	0	0	100
½ banana	.59	13.4	.27	58
1 teaspoon flaxseed oil	0	0	4.54	40
8 oz. of water				
Total calories				198
Total calories %	35	45	21	

Meal 5 (brown rice and chicken)	Protein	Carbohydrates	Fat	Calories
1 cup of broccoli	4.65	7.89	.55	43
1 cup long grain brown rice	5.04	45	1.76	216
6 oz. chicken breast	52.8	0	6.08	278
1 teaspoon olive oil	0	0	4.7	43
1 antioxidant				
Total calories				580
Total calories %	35	50	15	
Grand total calories				1500

Day 2

Meal 1 (cereal and milk)	Protein	Carbohydrates	Fat	Calories
1 cup of cereal multi grain	3.42	15.7	1.45	88
1 cup of organic milk 2%	8.13	11.7	4.68	121
1 multivitamin				
1 calcium/mag				
Total calories				209
Total calories %	22	52	26	

Meal 2 (protein drink)	Protein	Carbohydrates	Fat	Calories
1 scoop Gotein protein	12	2	0	55
1 cup of raspberries	1.12	14.1	.68	67
8 oz. soy milk	7	18	5	150
Total calories				272
Total calories %	29	50	18	
Meal 3 (turkey sandwich w/cheese)	Protein	Carbohydrates	Fat	Calories
2 slices of wheat bread	5.16	26.8	2.32	147
3 slices of turkey	21.4	.42	5.78	139
1 tablespoon low calorie mayonnaise	.05	2.5	3.0	36
1 slice of Swiss cheese	4	2	5	70
1 multivitamin				
1 calcium/mag				
Total calories				392
Total calories %	31	45	24	

Meal 4 (protein drink)	Protein	Carbohydrates	Fat	Calories
1 scoop Gotein protein	12	2	0	55
1 cup strawberries	.88	10.2	.53	49
8 oz. soy milk	7	18	5	150
Total calories				254
Total calories %	31	47	19	
Meal 5 (turkey meatloaf and sweet potatoes)	Protein	Carbohydrates	Fat	Calories
1 cup of green string beans	2.36	9.86	.35	52
1 cup of sweet potatoes	3.44	48.6	.22	206
4 oz. turkey meat loaf	22	0	1	100
1 teaspoon olive oil	0	0	4.7	43
1 antioxidant				
Total calories				401
Total calories %	28	47	23	
Grand total calories				1529

Day 3

Meal 1 (yogurt and granola)	Protein	Carbohydrates	Fat	Calories
1 oz. granola	2.9	19.1	4.9	126
6 oz. low fat yogurt	9	12.75	3	112
1 multivitamin				
1 calcium/mag				
Total calories				238
Total calories %	19	53	29	
Meal 2 (cottage cheese and fruit)	**Protein**	**Carbohydrates**	**Fat**	**Calories**
½ apple	.2	16.1	.38	68
1 piece bread rye	2.13	12.1	.83	64
1 tablespoon cream cheese	1.59	1.05	2.64	34
4 oz. cottage cheese	15.68	4.11	2.18	101
Total calories				269
Total calories %	29	49	20	

Meal 3 (pasta and chicken)	Protein	Carbohydrates	Fat	Calories
2 oz. tomato sauce	76	4.08	.10	20
1 cup pasta (whole wheat)	6.68	39.8	.94	197
3 oz. chicken breast	26.4	0	3.04	139
1 teaspoon olive oil	0	0	4.7	43
1 multivitamin				
1 calcium/mag				
Total calories				399
Total calories %	33	45	22	
Meal 4 (protein drink)	Protein	Carbohydrates	Fat	Calories
1 scoop Gotein protein	12	2	0	55
1 cup strawberries	.88	10.2	.53	49
8 oz. soy milk	7	18	5	150
Total calories				254
Total calories %	31	47	19	

Meal 5 (steak & yams)	Protein	Carbohydrates	Fat	Calories
1 cup yams	3.44	48.6	.22	206
3 oz. beef top round	27	0	4.17	153
1 tablespoon sour cream	1.2	1.81	0	10
1 antioxidant				
Total calories				369
Total calories %	34	55	11	
Grand total calories				1529

Day 4

Meal 1 (egg whites and wheat English muffin)	Protein	Carbohydrates	Fat	Calories
1 wheat English muffin	4.4	26.2	1.03	134
1 teaspoon butter	.04	0	3.83	34
½ slice of cheese	2	1	2.5	35
2 egg whites	7.38	.72	0	32
1 antioxidant				
1 calcium/mag				
Total calories				236
Total calories %	19	56	23	

Meal 2 (protein drink)	Protein	Carbohydrates	Fat	Calories
1 scoop Gotein protein	12	2	0	55
1 cup strawberries	.88	10.2	.53	49
1 teaspoon flaxseed oil	0	0	4.54	40
8 oz. water				
Total calories				189
Total calories %	51	27	21	

Meal 3 (tuna pita pocket)	Protein	Carbohydrates	Fat	Calories
1 pear	.65	24.2	.66	98
1 piece of wheat pita	5.46	33.4	.72	165
3 oz. tuna fish in water	22.7	0	2.09	116
1 tablespoon low calorie mayonnaise	.05	2.5	3	36
1 multivitamin				
1 calcium/mag				
Total calories				415
Total calories %	27	58	14	

Meal 4 (protein drink)	Protein	Carbohydrates	Fat	Calories
1 scoop Gotein protein	25	0	0	100
1 cup strawberries	.88	10.2	.53	58
1 teaspoon flaxseed oil	0	0	4.54	40
8 oz. water				
Total calories				198
Total calories %	51	27	21	
Meal 5 (red snapper and mixed veggies)	Protein	Carbohydrates	Fat	Calories
4 oz. mixed veggies	3.24	14.82	.17	66
1 cup brown rice	5.04	45.0	1.76	216
3 oz. red snapper	20.88	0	1.36	95
1 teaspoon olive oil	0	0	4.7	43
1 antioxidant				
Total calories				420
Total calories %	25	61	12	
Grand total calories				1458

Day 5

Meal 1 (cereal; and milk)	Protein	Carbohydrates	Fat	Calories
1 cup whole grain cereal	3.3	26	.69	123
1 cup organic milk 2%	8.13	11.7	4.68	121
1 multivitamin				
1 calcium/mag				
Total calories				244
Total calories %	21	55	24	
Meal 2 (protein shake)	Protein	Carbohydrates	Fat	Calories
1 scoop Gotein protein	12	2	0	55
1 cup blueberries	.88	10.2	.53	49
8 oz. of soy milk	7	18	5	150
Total calories				254
Total calories %	31	47	19	

Meal 3 (shrimp over salad)	Protein	Carbohydrates	Fat	Calories
1 tbs. low cal French dressing	0	2.1	2.5	31
1 cup broccoli	4.65	7.89	.55	43
1 cup cauliflower	2.3	5.1	.56	28
2 cups salad romaine	.2.54	10	.7	49
½ cup boiled corn	2.72	20.6	1.05	102
3 oz. large shrimp	17.94	1.33	1.56	88
1 multivitamin				
1 calcium/mag				
Total calories	.			344
Total calories %	35	54	18	
Meal 4 (protein drink)	Protein	Carbohydrates	Fat	Calories
1 scoop Gotein protein	12	2	0	55
1 cup raspberries	.88	10.2	.53	49
8 oz. soy milk	7	18	5	150
Total calories	.			254
Total calories %	31	47	19	

Meal 5 (salmon and yams)	Protein	Carbohydrates	Fat	Calories
1 cup green peas	2.36	9.86	.35	52
1 cup yams	3.44	48.6	.22	206
3 oz. salmon	21.6	0	6.9	154
1 teaspoon butter	.04	0	3.83	34
1 antioxidant				
Total calories				447
Total calories %	24	52	22	
Grand total calories				1544

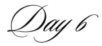

Day 6

Meal 1 (oatmeal w/soymilk)	Protein	Carbohydrates	Fat	Calories
1 cup oatmeal	9.12	37.96	3.52	217
8 oz. soy milk	7	18	5	150
1 multivitamin				
1 calcium/mag				
Total calories				367
Total calories %	24	53	23	

Meal 2 (protein drink)	Protein	Carbohydrates	Fat	Calories
1 scoop Gotein protein	12	2	0	55
1 cup blueberries	.97	20.4	.55	81
1 teaspoon flaxseed oil	0	0	4.54	40
8 oz. of water				
Total calories	.			176
Total calories %	29	50	25	

Meal 3 (chicken tortilla)	Protein	Carbohydrates	Fat	Calories
2 cups broccoli	9.3	15.78	1.09	87
2 cups romaine salad	2.54	10	.7	49
2 tablespoons salsa	1.51	8.15	.19	40
1 corn tortilla	1.71	14	.75	66
2 oz. chicken breast	18.48	0	2.13	97
1 teaspoon olive oil	0	0	4.7	43
1 multivitamin				
1 calcium/mag				
Total calories	.			384
Total calories %	34	49	22	

Meal 4 (protein drink)	Protein	Carbohydrates	Fat	Calories
1 scoop Gotein protein	12	2	0	55
1 cup strawberries	.88	10.2	.53	49
1 teaspoon flaxseed oil	0	0	4.54	40
8 oz. of water				
Total calories	.	50	15	144
Total calories %	35	33	31	

Meal 5 (pasta and chicken)	Protein	Carbohydrates	Fat	Calories
1 cup kale	2.36	9.86	.35	52
1 cup pasta any kind	11.19	55.8	1.13	261
2 oz. chicken breast	18.48	0	2.13	97
1 teaspoon olive oil	0	0	4.7	43
1 antioxidant				
Total calories				453
Total calories %	28	57	16	
Grand total calories				1525

Day 7

Meal 1 (eggs and toast)	Protein	Carbohydrates	Fat	Calories
2 slices whole wheat bread	5.16	26.8	2.32	147
1 slice cheese	4	2	5	70
2 egg whites	7.38	.72	0	32
1 multivitamin				
1 calcium/mag				
Total calories				250
Total calories %	27	47	25	

Meal 2 (protein drink)	Protein	Carbohydrates	Fat	Calories
1 scoop Gotein protein	12	2	0	55
1 cup blueberries	.49	10.2	.28	40
8 oz. soy milk	7	18	5	150
Total calories	.			245
Total calories %	29	50	18	

Meal 3 (turkey sandwich)	Protein	Carbohydrates	Fat	Calories
1 orange	1.23	15.5	.16	68
2 slices wheat bread	5.16	26.8	2.32	147
2 oz. turkey breast	15.42	0	.60	67
1 teaspoon mayonnaise	.05	.12	3.67	33
1 multivitamin				
1 calcium/mag				
Total calories				316
Total calories %	27	53	19	
Meal 4 (protein drink)	Protein	Carbohydrates	Fat	Calories
1 scoop Gotein protein	12	2	0	55
1 cup strawberries	.88	10.2	.53	49
8 oz. soy milk	7	18	5	150
Total calories				254
Total calories %	31	47	19	

Meal 5 (chicken and rice)	Protein	Carbohydrates	Fat	Calories
1 cup brown rice	5.04	45.00	1.76	216
¼ cup black beans	3.83	10.1	.22	56
3 oz. chicken breast	26.4	0	3.04	139
1 teaspoon olive oil	0	0	4.7	43
1 antioxidant				
Total calories				454
Total calories %	28	53	15	
Grand total calories				1519

The Wedding Workout at Three Months

In these next three months, you will change your training routine. These changes are necessary to force your body to continuously adapt to the workload. As you raise the activity bar you will feel challenged, which will prevent you from getting bored.

Focus on the following list as you adjust your workout for the next three months:

- Keep it intense. Each time you reduce your caloric intake you will not have as much energy as before. At first, you might not be able to do as many sets. You must still train with maximum intensity and take every set to failure so that you do not lose precious muscle tissue.

- Change the resting periods. Reduce the rest time from 30 seconds to 15 seconds for every aspect of the workout.

- Do not change the order of the exercises. The order matters.

- Change your weights. You should be adding weight when you can perform the highest number of repetitions in the first set in perfect form. If you are doing three sets of 15, 12, 10 repetitions, and you can do them perfectly with 10-pound dumbbells on the first set, it is time to increase to 15-pound dumbbells.

- Work out more often. You will still be strength training fours days per week. Now, add an extra day of aerobic, abs, stretching work. Your schedule should now look like the following:

Day 1: 1 hour

Day 2: 1 hour

Day 3: Rest

Day 4: 1 hour

Day 5: 1 hour

Day 6: 35 minutes (Aerobic training, abdominal work, and stretching only)

Day 7: Rest

The Gym Workout

Daily Warm-Ups

Heart rate: 60% of maximum heart rate

Duration: 5 minutes

Begin with a light aerobic workout, which should be done at 60 percent your maximum heart rate. Choose from the following activities:

- Treadmill
- Recumbent bicycle
- Stair climber
- Elliptical climber

Remember to use your heart rate monitor. Monitor your heart rate closely.

Dynamic Stretch

Heart rate:60 % of maximum heart rate

Duration: 5 minutes

Warm-Ups

- Prisoner Squats: 3 sets of 20 repetitions, page 50
- Single-Leg Squat Touchdown: 3 sets, 15 repetitions each leg, page 50
- Arm Circles: 2 sets, 40 seconds each arm in each direction, page 50
- Plank Posture with Downward Facing Dog: 10 repetitions of the full cycle, page 51
- Medicine Ball Rotations: 15 full rotations, page 52

Progress from one exercise to the next without resting in between. Repeat the entire circuit twice before moving to the abdominal drills.

Abdominal Drills

Heart rate: 55% of maximum heart rate

Duration: 5 minutes

In the three-month workout, the abdominal drills change. Now you will do three sets of 20 repetitions of each exercise. Complete one set of each exercise in the routine as a circuit before beginning the second set. Rest 15 seconds between sets. The first three days of abdominal workouts target a particular part of the torso. The last day is a combination workout. Remember to stretch your abdominal muscles either over a physioball or do a yoga Cobra Posture (see page 56) as a warm-up for your abs before these routines. On Day 6, repeat Abdominal Group 1.

Abdominal Group 1 (Upper Abdominals)

- Machine Crunch, page 82
- Butterfly Crunch, page 63
- Cable Crunch with Rope, page 81

Abdominal Group 2 (Lower Abdominals)

- Reverse Crunch on Incline Board, page 84
- Hanging Run-in-Place, page 80
- Vertical Bench Leg Raise, page 79

Abdominal Group 3 (Obliques)

- Decline Bench Twisting Crunch, page 78
- Hanging Knee Raise to the Side, page 83
- Bicycle, see page 70

Abdominal Group 4 (Complete Abdominal Workout: Upper, Lower, Obliques)

- Decline-Bench Twisting Crunch, page 78
- Figure Four Crunch, page 72
- Cross Over Split Leg Crunch, page 62

Strength Training

Heart rate: 65 % of maximum heart rate

Duration: 20 minutes

In the three-month workout, you will be swapping two days of exercises. Remember to train with intensity and increase the weights on all exercises as needed. Also, do not change the order of the exercises. The order matters. On your fifth day of exercise, repeat Strength Training Group 1.

Strength Training Group 1

- Hack Squats: 2 sets, 20 repetitions, page 108
- Smith Machine Reverse Lunges: 2 sets, 15 repetitions, page 104
- Abductor Machine: 3 sets, 15 repetitions, page 113
- Bent-Over Dumbbell Rows: 2 sets, 12 repetitions, page 136
- Good Morning: 2 sets, 12 repetitions, page 137
- Incline Dumbbell Press: 2 sets, 12 repetitions, page 128
- Flat Dumbbell Flyes: 2 sets, 10 repetitions, page 125
- Rear Deltoid Flyes: 2 sets, 10 repetitions, page 91
- Bench Dips: 2 sets, 15 repetitions, page 90
- Two Arm High Cable Curl: 2 sets, 12 repetitions, page 100
- Seated Calf Raise: 2 sets, 15 repetitions, page 94

Strength Training Group 2

- Leg Press: 3 sets, 15 repetitions, page 93
- Seated Leg Curl: 2 sets ,12 repetitions, page 95
- Leg Extension: 2 sets, 15 repetitions, page 105

- Seated Machine Press: 2 sets, 12 repetitions, page 115
- Pec Dec 3 sets: 15 repetitions, page 106
- Shoulder Press Machine: 3 sets, 15 repetitions, page 116
- Triceps Pressdown: 3 sets, 15 repetitions, page 98
- Hammer Curls: 2 sets, 15 repetitions, page 152
- Standing Calf Raise: 3 sets, 15 repetitions, page 96

Strength Training Group 3

- Lying Leg Curl: 2 sets, first 20, then 15 repetitions each, page 92
- Smith Machine Squats: 2 sets: 15 repetitions each, page 103
- Adductor Machine: 2 sets, 15 repetitions, page 113
- Assisted Pullup Machine: 2 sets, 15 repetitions each, page 119
- Rear Deltoid Flyes: 3 sets: 15, 12, and 10 repetitions each, page 91
- Side Lateral Raises: 2 sets, 15, then 12 repetitions each, page 147
- Lying Triceps Barbell Extension: 2 sets, first set 15, then 12, page 118
- Close Grip Bench Press: 2 sets, 15 repetitions, page 120

- One Arm Preacher Dumbbell Curls: 2 sets, 10 repetitions each, page 123
- Leg Press Calf Raise: 2 sets, 15 repetitions each, page 93

Strength Training Group 4

- Leg Extensions: 2 sets, 15 repetitions, page 105
- Seated Leg Curls: 3 sets, 15, 12, and 10 repetitions each, page 95
- Barbell Lunges: 3 sets, 15 repetitions each, page 109
- Cable Crossover: 3 sets, 15 repetitions each, page 102
- Seated Cable Rows: 2 sets, 15 repetitions each, page 97
- Wide Grip Front Pulldown: 2 sets, 15 repetitions each, page 117
- Upright Rows: 2 sets, first set 15, then 12 repetitions, page 144
- Overhead Rope Extension: 2 sets, 15, then 12 repetitions, page 101
- Standing Barbell Curls: 3 sets, 15 repetitions each, page 111
- Standing Calf Raise: 2 sets, 15 repetitions each, page 96

Aerobic Workout

Heart rate: 75-80% of maximum heart rate

Duration: 20 minutes

For the three-month program, choose two pieces of equipment for each week. Sticking with the same gym equipment day after day will lead to boredom. Worse yet, your exercise may become inefficient, and it is likely that you will hit a plateau. You will burn more calories if you rotate machines between the stair climber, treadmill, elliptical climber, recumbent bike, etc.

For example, the Week 1 workout should feature the stair climber and the treadmill. Skip the running if you have knee or lower back injuries, and walk instead. The following week, choose two different pieces of equipment, like a stationary bike and the elliptical climber. The next week, vary with the stair climber and the bike, etc. This should keep you interested for the duration of the program.

If you've been exercising regularly, following the six-month workout, your endurance level should be pretty darn good. You should be challenging yourself every week by increasing your intensity level. Monitor your heart rate closely. If your heart rate is too low you are not training hard enough. Stay focused and push yourself, but know your limitations. Continue to do your extra day of aerobic work, abdominals, and post workout stretch on Day 6.

First Piece of Equipment: Stair climber

Duration: 10 minutes

Tip: Increase the intensity level every 1 minute.

Duration in minutes	Description	Maximum Heart Rate
1	warm-up	60%
1	low intensity	60%
1	medium intensity	70%
1	high intensity	80%
1	high intensity	80%
1	recovery	60%
1	medium intensity	70%
1	high intensity	80%
1	high intensity	80%
1	medium intensity	65%

Change Equipment: Elliptical climber

Duration: 10 minutes

Tip: Increase the intensity level every 2 minutes.

Duration in minutes	Description	Maximum Heart Rate
2	medium intensity	70%
2	medium intensity	70%
2	high intensity	80%
2	high intensity	80%
2	cool down	60%

Cool-Down Workout Stretching:

Heart rate: 50% of maximum heart rate

Duration: 5 minutes

You have now completed another good workout. The three-month workout features a new routine of post workout stretches. Remember to listen to your body during stretching, and be aware of any discomfort you might feel. Never continue an uncomfortable stretch!

- Wall Stretch, page 159
- Head Lean, page 159
- Jaw Tuck, page 160
- Back Reach, page 160
- Wrist Stretch, page 160
- Bent Knee Lunge, page 161
- Hamstring Stretch, page 161
- Lateral Stride, page 162
- Spine Rotation, page 162
- Wall Stretch, page 163

At-home Program

You will be able to complete all of these exercises without using gym equipment. Make sure to include every aspect of the Bootcamp workout in your at home routine. The time commitments also remain the same. The Dynamic Stretch and Post Workout Stretch in this section are exactly the same as the gym version.

Abdominal Drills

Heart rate: 55% maximum heart rate

Duration: 5 minutes

In the three month workout you will do three sets of 20 repetitions of each exercise. Complete one set of each exercise in the routine as a circuit before beginning the second set. Rest only 15 seconds between sets. The first three days of the ab workouts target particular part of the torso. The last day is a combination workout. Remember to stretch your abdominal muscles either over a physioball or do a yoga Cobra Posture before the abdominal drills to warm up.

Abdominal Group 1 at Home
(Upper Abdominals)

- Figure-Four Crunch, page 72
- Butterfly Crunch, page 63
- Thigh Slide Crunch, page 64

Abdominal Group 2 at Home
(Lower Abdominals)

- Scissors Kick, page 66
- Bent-Leg Hip Raise, page 69
- Reverse Crunch with Physioball, page 75

Abdominal Group 3 at Home (obliques)

- Twisting Crunch on the Physioball, page 73
- Side Bend, page 67
- Side Jackknife, page 76

Abdominal Group 4 at Home
(Complete Abdominal
Workout—Upper, Lower, Obliques)

- Hands Over Head Crunch, page 71
- Hip Thrust, page 74
- Cross Over Split Leg Crunch, page 62
- Bicycle, page 70

Strength Training

Heart rate: 65% of maximum heart rate

Duration: 20 minutes

There are four new strength-training routines in the three-month workout. Follow the routines in the order listed. Remember to train with intensity and increase the weight on all exercises.

Strength Training Group 1 at Home

- Stiff-Leg Deadlift: 2 sets, 15 repetitions, page 133
- Glute Lifts with Physioball: 2 sets, 15 repetitions, page 149
- Good Morning: 2 sets, 12 repetitions, page 137
- Physioball Push-Ups 2 sets: 10 repetitions, page 150
- Upright Rows: 3 sets, 12 repetitions, page 144
- Bent Over Lateral Raise: 3 sets, 12 repetitions, page 131
- Seated Overhead Dumbbell Extension: 2 sets, 12 repetitions, page 153
- Standing Dumbbell Curls: 2 sets, 12 repetitions, page 140
- Standing One Leg Calf Raise: 2 sets, 15 repetitions, page 135

Strength Training Group 2 at Home

- Alternating Dumbbell Lunges: 3 sets, 15 repetitions, page 142
- Physioball Dumbbell Squat: 3 sets, 15 repetitions, page 132
- Bent Over Dumbbell Rows: 2 sets, 12 repetitions, page 136
- Flat Dumbbell Press: 3 sets, 12 repetitions, page 110
- Overhead Lateral Raise: 2 sets, 12 repetitions, page 143
- Shrugs: 2 sets, 12 repetitions, page 152
- Chair Dips: 2 sets, 15 repetitions, page 139
- Dumbbell Concentration Curls: 2 sets, 15 repetitions, page 126
- Standing One-Leg Calf Raise: 2 sets, 15 repetitions, page 135

Strength Training Group 3 at Home

- Leg Lifts: 3 sets, 15 each, page 148
- Glute Lifts With Physioball: 2 sets: 20 repetitions each, page 149
- Dumbbell Squats: 2 sets, 15 repetitions each, page 141
- Push-Ups on Physioball: 2 sets, 10 repetitions each, page 150

- Side Lateral Raise: 2 sets, 15 then 12 repetitions each, page 147
- Physioball One-Arm Dumbbell Extensions: 2 sets, 15 repetitions each, page 134
- Hammer Curls: 2 sets, 15 repetitions each, page 151
- Standing One-Leg Calf Raise: 3 sets, 15 repetitions each, page 135

Strength Training Group 4 at Home

- Stiff-Leg Deadlift: 3 sets, 10 repetitions each, page 133
- Bent-Over Dumbbell Rows: 3 sets, first set 15, then 12 repetitions each, page 136
- Flat Dumbbell Press: 3 sets, first set 15, then 12 repetitions, page 110
- Side Lateral Raise: 2 sets, 15 repetitions each, page 147
- Shrugs: 3 sets, 15 repetitions, page 152
- Seated Overhead Dumbbell Extension: 3 sets, 15 repetitions each, page 153
- Standing Dumbbell Curls: 3 sets, 15 repetitions each, page 140
- Dumbbell Concentration Curls: 2 sets, 15 repetitions, page 126
- Standing One-Leg Calf Raise: 2 sets, 15 repetitions each, page 135

Aerobic Workout:
High-intensity Interval Training

Heart rate: 75 to 80% of maximum heart rate

Duration: 20 minutes

To add variety to your at-home cardiovascular workout, jump rope for 10 minutes and then perform 10 push-ups. Keep repeating the cycle for 20 minutes.

If you do in-line skating or have a traditional bike, stick with one or the other for 20 minutes. No matter what you choose, be sure to check your heart rate so that you are training between 75 percent to percent of your maximum heart rate. Continue to do your extra day of aerobic work, abdominal drills, and post workout stretching on Day 6.

Post Workout Stretching:

Heart rate: 50% of maximum heart rate

Duration: 5 minutes

You have now completed another good workout. The three-month workout features a new routine of post workout stretches. Remember to listen to your body during stretching, and be aware of any discomfort you might feel. Never continue an uncomfortable stretch!

- Wall Stretch, page 159
- Head Lean, page 159
- Jaw Tuck, page 160
- Back Reach, page 160
- Wrist Stretch, page 160
- Bent Knee Lunge, page 161
- Hamstring Stretch, page 161
- Lateral Stride, page 162
- Spine Rotation, page 162
- Wall Stretch, page 163

Take Time Off!

Congratulations! You have completed the second part of the Bridal Bootcamp™ Fitness program. It's time to take off another five days. Do absolutely nothing. Start getting excited: your big day is only a month away!

CHAPTER SEVEN:

One Month to the Wedding

I f you've made it this far, you are probably looking and feeling great. By following the eating plan and exercising regularly, you should see significant changes in your body. Your clothes should feel looser all over. Even your wedding dress might have to be taken down one or two whole sizes!

Have you noticed that these physical alterations are accompanied by profound lifestyle changes? At night, you might find that you can stay up later than before and still sleep soundly. Your overall energy level may have increased so that you wake up feeling refreshed, and stay alert for longer periods during the day. You might have thought that this was due to all the excitement of the wedding, but it isn't. You've created a whole new you: you are reaching your physical potential.

If you haven't been as diligent as you wanted to be, now is the time to really work. You can't completely make up for lost time, but this month will prove to be the toughest part of the program. If you follow these guidelines, you should see results quickly. If you can stick with the program, you can make changes that will last a lifetime. So get focused, because we have the last pounds of fat to shed.

Take another set of photographs, (front, side,

and rear shots of your body) and compare them to the two previous sets in your journal. Take your girth measurements, and compare the totals as well as the individual measurements. Don't forget to weigh, and use the skinfold caliper to measure your body fat, every other week.

If you are not at your goal weight, reduce your calories by 10 percent.

Earlier, we determined that Carol's new caloric maintenance level was 1500. We deducted 20 percent from 1800, her previous daily calorie allowance. Two months later, she now weighs 135 pounds. The first three months she lost 15 pounds, the following two months she lost 10 pounds. If you are like Carol, you'll see that your results at the beginning of the program were the most dramatic, but slow down as your body adjusts to the reduction in calories you are consuming. But do not fret, you will still be able to reach your fitness goals. You just have to be patient and continue the protocols.

Carol needs to recalculate her new daily calorie allotment. Remember, her goal is to weigh 130 pounds for her wedding, so she needs to lose an additional 5 pounds. She has only three weeks left before the wedding, and it's crunch time.

Carol daily calorie allotment is 1500 calories.
1500 - 10% = 1350 (round out to 1300)

Carol's new daily caloric allotment is 1300 calories.

What to Eat

Each day on the three-month meal plan is roughly 1300 calories. Refer back to your weight loss caloric intake number in your journal. If your number is less than 1300 calories, you will need to modify the meals accordingly to your assigned caloric intake number. You can remove some food items throughout the day until you reach your number, but don't skip any of the meals entirely.

For the first week, follow the meal plans exactly. Afterward, you can create your own 1300 calorie days from the sample meals. Use the guidelines to show how to mix the appropriate four groups to get to the proper ratio of 50 percent carbohydrates, 30 percent protein, 20 percent fat.

1300 CALORIE MEAL PLAN

Continue to eat low glycemic carbohydrates. You will continue to do this until the week before the wedding. Keep your water intake high and continue to follow the plan until the big day.

Meal 1 (cereal and milk)	Protein	Carbohydrates	Fat	Calories
1 cups whole grain cereal	3.42	15.7	1.45	88
½ cup low fat milk, 2%	4.07	5.85	2.34	60
1 multivitamin				
1 calcium/mag				
Total calories				149
Total calories %	20	57	22	

Meal 2 (green salad with turkey slices)	Protein	Carbohydrates	Fat	Calories
1 cup broccoli	4.65	7.89	.55	43
2 cups lettuce	2.54	10.	.7	49
½ cantaloupe	2.34	22.4	.75	105
2 slices turkey breast	10.7	.21	2.89	69
1 tbs. oil & vinegar dressing	0	1.7	3	34
Total calories				302
Total calories %	26	55	23	
Meal 3 (pasta and chicken)	Protein	Carbohydrates	Fat	Calories
1 cup broccoli	4.65	7.89	.55	43
1 cup pasta whole wheat	6.68	39.8	.94	197
2 oz. chicken breast	18.48	0	2.13	97
1 teaspoon olive oil	0	0	4.7	43
1 multivitamin				
1 calcium/mag				
Total calories				381
Total calories %	31	50	19	

Meal 4 (eggs and wheat bread)	Protein	Carbohydrates	Fat	Calories
2 slices of wheat bread	4.36	24.8	1.95	130
1 teaspoon butter	.04	0	3.83	34
2 egg whites	7.38	.72	0	32
Total calories				196
Total calories %	26	55	19	
Meal 5 (beef and barley)	Protein	Carbohydrates	Fat	Calories
½ cup barley	7.00	41.6	1.4	200
2 oz. beef	18.00	0	2.78	102
1 antioxidant				
Total calories				302
Total calories %	33	55	12	
Grand total calories				1331

Day 2

Meal 1 (oatmeal)	Protein	Carbohydrates	Fat	Calories
1 cup oatmeal	7.11	29.61	2.75	169
1 cup 2% milk	8.13	11.7	4.68	121
1 multivitamin				
1 calcium/mag				
Total calories				290
Total calories %	20	56	22	
Meal 2 (chicken and brown rice)	Protein	Carbohydrates	Fat	Calories
1 cup brown rice	5.04	45.	1.76	216
2 oz. chicken breast	17.69	0	2.04	93
Total calories				309
Total calories %	32	55	13	

Meal 3 (tuna sandwich)	Protein	Carbohydrates	Fat	Calories
2 piece whole wheat bread	5.16	26.8	2.32	147
2 oz. tuna fish in water	15.89	0	1.46	81
1 multivitamin				
1 calcium/mag				
Total calories				228
Total calories %	35	47	18	
Meal 4 (lentil soup)	Protein	Carbohydrates	Fat	Calories
1 piece whole grain bread	3.08	18.2	1.05	95
8 oz. lentil soup	7.0	9.0	1.0	70
1 tsp. butter	.04	0	3.83	34
Total calories				200
Total calories %	20	54	26	

Meal 5 (turkey and sweet potatoes)	Protein	Carbohydrates	Fat	Calories
½ cup of sweet potato	.98	13.85	.06	58
½ cup rice pudding	3	20	3	120
2 oz. ground turkey	11.0	0	.5	50
1 tsp. butter	.04	0	3.83	34
1 antioxidant				
Total calories				262
Total calories %	22	51	25	
Grand total calories				1289

Day 3

Meal 1 (oatbran & soy milk)	Protein	Carbohydrates	Fat	Calories
1 cup oat bran	8	23	4	140
1 cup soy milk	7	18	5	150
1 multivitamin				
1 calcium/mag				
Total calories				290
Total calories %	17	54	39	

Meal 2 (split pea soup)	Protein	Carbohydrates	Fat	Calories
12 oz. split pea soup	10.83	32.1	2.22	186
1 tsp. flaxseed oil	0	0	4.54	40
Total calories				226
Total calories %	19	56	26	

Meal 3 (chicken sandwich)	Protein	Carbohydrates	Fat	Calories
1 tangerine	.53	9.41	.16	37
2 slices of wheat bread	5.16	26.8	2.32	147
2 oz. chicken breast	18.48	0	2.13	139
1 tbs. low calorie mayonnaise	.05	2.5	3	36
1 multivitamin				
1 calcium/mag				
Total calories				317
Total calories %	30	48	21	

Meal 4 (tuna tortilla)	Protein	Carbohydrates	Fat	Calories
½ grapefruit	.6	11.9	.1	46
1 corn tortilla	1.71	14	.75	66
2 oz. tuna in water	15.89	0	1.46	81
1 tbs. low calorie mayonnaise	.05	2.5	3	36
Total calories				229
Total calories %	31	49	20	
Meal 5 (pasta and ground turkey)	Protein	Carbohydrates	Fat	Calories
1 cup string beans	2.36	9.86	.35	52
½ cup pasta	3.73	18.6	.38	87
2 oz. ground turkey	11	0	.5	50
1 tsp. olive oil	0	0	4.7	43
1 antioxidant				
Total calories				232
Total calories %	29	49	22	
Grand total calories				1295

Day 4

Meal 1 (pancake and eggs)	Protein	Carbohydrates	Fat	Calories
1 tablespoon low calorie maple syrup	0	13.4	.04	53
1 pancake (whole grain)	2.13	7.0	2.05	56
3 egg whites	9.84	.96	0	43
1 multivitamin				
1 calcium/mag				
Total calories				152
Total calories %	30	55	15	
Meal 2 (rice, beans and chicken)	Protein	Carbohydrates	Fat	Calories
1 cup string beans	2.36	9.86	.35	52
½ cup brown rice	2.52	22.5	.88	108
¼ cup beans	3.83	10.1	.22	56
2 oz. chicken breast	18.48	0	2.13	97
1 teaspoon flaxseed oil	0	0	4.54	40
Total calories				353
Total calories %	33	47	20	

Meal 3 (roast beef sandwich)	Protein	Carbohydrates	Fat	Calories
2 slices whole grain bread	5.16	26.8	.32	147
2 slices roast beef	21.3	0	4.68	132
1 tbs. mustard	.06	.50	.99	10
1 multivitamin				
1 calcium/mag				
Total calories				289
Total calories %	28	48	24	
Meal 4 (oatmeal and soymilk)	Protein	Carbohydrates	Fat	Calories
1 cup oatmeal	4.56	18.98	1.76	108
1 cup soy milk	7	18	5	150
Total calories				258
Total calories %	22	54	24	

Meal 5 (catfish and brown rice)	Protein	Carbohydrates	Fat	Calories
1 cup brown rice	5.04	45	1.76	216
3 oz. fish-catfish	19.3	0	4.53	123
1 antioxidant				
Total calories				339
Total calories %	28	53	19	
Grand total calories				1391

Day 5

Meal 1 (eggs and 7 grain bread)	Protein	Carbohydrates	Fat	Calories
2 pieces 7 grain bread	5.88	30.4	.82	143
1 teaspoon butter	.04	0	3.83	34
2 egg whites	7.38	.72	0	32
1 multivitamin				
1 calcium/mag				
Total calories				210
Total calories %	25	59	16	

Meal 2 (turkey and Caesar salad)	Protein	Carbohydrates	Fat	Calories
2 cups lettuce	2.54	10	.7	49
1 tomato	1.05	5.71	.41	25
½ cup yams	1.72	24.3	.11	103
2 oz. turkey breast	14.07	0	.84	69
1 tbs. Caesar dressing	0	1	7	70
Total calories				317
Total calories %	24	51	25	
Meal 3 (ham sandwich)	Protein	Carbohydrates	Fat	Calories
2 pieces pumpernickel bread	5.56	30.4	1.98	160
2 slices of ham	14.91	0	3.28	92
1 multivitamin				
1 calcium/mag				
Total calories				252
Total calories %	32	48	20	

Meal 4 (protein drink)	Protein	Carbohydrates	Fat	Calories
1 scoop Gotein protein	12	2	0	55
½ cup blueberries	.49	0	.28	40
1 cup soy milk	7	18	5	150
Total calories				245
Total calories %	31	49	20	
Meal 5 (pasta and ground turkey)	Protein	Carbohydrates	Fat	Calories
¼ cup green peas	2.15	6.25	.09	33
½ cup whole wheat pasta	3.34	19.9	.47	98
4 oz. ground turkey	22.0	0	1.0	100
1 tsp. flaxseed oil	0	0	4.54	40
1 antioxidant				
Total calories				272
Total calories %	25	53	22	
Grand total calories				1296

Day 6

Meal 1 (apple and cottage cheese)	Protein	Carbohydrates	Fat	Calories
½ apple	.2	16.1	.38	68
3 oz. 2% cottage cheese	11.76	3.08	1.64	76
1 multivitamin				
1 calcium/mag				
Total calories				144
Total calories %	33	52	12	

Meal 2 (brown rice and turkey)	Protein	Carbohydrates	Fat	Calories
1 cup cauliflower	2.3	5.1	.56	28
1 cup brown rice	5.04	45	1.76	216
2 oz. turkey breast	17.99	0	.7	78
1 teaspoon olive oil	0	0	4.7	43
Total calories				365
Total calories %	28	54	18	

Meal 3 (salad and ham pita pocket	Protein	Carbohydrates	Fat	Calories
½ cucumber	1.04	4.17	0	19
2 cups lettuce	2.54	10	.7	49
1 whole wheat pita	4.4	24.8	1.16	120
2 slices of ham	6.2	0	4.66	65
Balsamic vinegar	0	0	0	0
1 multivitamin				
1 calcium/mag				
Total calories				253
Total calories %	28	54	18	
Meal 4 (protein drink)	Protein	Carbohydrates	Fat	Calories
1 scoop Gotein protein	12	2	0	55
1 cup strawberries	.88	10.2	.53	49
1 cup vanilla soy milk	7	18	5	150
Total calories				254
Total calories %	31	47	22	

Meal 5 (tuna pita pocket)	Protein	Carbohydrates	Fat	Calories
1 tbs. dressing low calorie Italian	0	1	2	22
1 cup salad	1.27	5	.35	24
1 tomato	1.05	5.71	.41	25
1 whole wheat pita pocket	4.4	24.8	1.16	120
2 oz. tuna fish in water	15.89	0	1.46	81
1 antioxidant				
Total calories				272
Total calories %	33	53	14	
Grand total calories				1288

Meal 1 (whole grain cereal)	Protein	Carbohydrates	Fat	Calories
1 cup whole grain cereal	2.76	23.1	.49	107
1 cup 2% milk	8.13	11.7	4.68	121
1 multivitamin				
1 calcium/mag				
Total calories				228
Total calories %	25	54	21	
Meal 2 (yogurt and fruit)	Protein	Carbohydrates	Fat	Calories
½ medium orange	.62	7.75	.08	34
8 oz. low fat yogurt	9	12.75	3	112
Total calories				146
Total calories %	26	55	19	

Meal 3 (salmon and brown rice)	Protein	Carbohydrates	Fat	Calories
8 oz. vegetable juice	1.52	11	22	46
1 cup brown rice	2.52	22.5	.88	108
2.5 oz. salmon	18.0	0	5.75	128
1 multivitamin				
1 calcium/mag				
Total calories				283
Total calories %	30	50	20	
Meal 4 (rice cakes & yogurt)	Protein	Carbohydrates	Fat	Calories
1 tbs peanut butter	4.5	3	8	95
2 rice cakes plain	1.47	15.33	.63	73
8 oz. yogurt	13.0	17	.36	120
Total calories				320
Total calories %	27	48	25	

Meal 5 (rice and chicken with veggies)	Protein	Carbohydrates	Fat	Calories
1 cup broccoli	4.65	7.89	.55	43
1 cup brown rice	5.04	45	1.76	216
2 oz. chicken breast	18.48	0	2.13	97
1 teaspoon olive oil	0	0	4.54	40
1 antioxidant				
Total calories				396
Total calories %	30	49	21	
Grand total calories				1373

The Wedding Workout At One Month

In the one-month final crunch you will add another day of twenty minutes of cardiovascular interval training. You'll be training six days per week, and your schedule should look like the following:

Day 1: 1 hour

Day 2: 1 hour

Day 3: Rest

Day 4: 1 hour

Day 5: 1 hour

Day 6: 35 minutes (Aerobic training, abdominal drills, and post workout stretch)

Day 7: 35 minutes (Aerobic training, abdominal drills, and post workout stretch)

Continue for three weeks. A week before your wedding, stop. Let yourself relax, and enjoy your last week of single life. It's time to give your body a rest. Relax and de-stress.

One Month in the Gym

Before you begin the program, put on your heart monitor!

Warm-Up

Heart rate: 60% of your maximum heart rate

Duration: 5 minutes

Begin with light cardiovascular work which should be done at 65 percent your maximum heart rate. Choose from the following activities, and set a timer for a five-minute warm-up routine:

- Treadmill
- Recumbent bicycle
- Stair climber
- Elliptical climber

Dynamic Stretch

Heart rate:60% of your maximum heart rate

Duration: 5 minutes

Perform this circuit 3 times, resting only a maximum of 30 seconds between sets.

- Starburst: see page 53
- Kick-Out with Jumping Jacks: see page 53

- Jumping Squats: see page 54
- Hip Swing: see page 54

Abdominal Drills

Heart rate: 55% of maximum heart rate

Durations: 5 minutes

Choose two exercises from each group: upper, lower, and obliques. **Do 2 sets of 25 repetitions of each exercise.** Complete all of the sets for that exercise before you proceed to the next. Cut down your rest period to only 5 seconds between exercises. Remember to stretch your abdominal muscles either over a physioball or do a yoga Cobra Posture before doing the following routines.

Abdominal Group 1 (Upper Abdominals)
- Cross Over Split Leg Crunch, page 62
- Machine Crunch, page 82
- Cable Crunch with Rope, page 81

Abdominal Group 2 (Obliques)
- Bicycle, page 70
- Side Bend, page 67
- Oblique Crunch, page 60

Abdominal Group 1 (Lower Abdominals)
- Double Crunch, page 61
- Reverse Crunch on Incline Board, page 84
- Vertical Bench Leg Raise, page 79

Strength Training

Heart rate: 65% of maximum heart rate

Duration: 20 minutes

Remember to train with intensity and increase the weight on all exercises. Perform one exercise after the other. As before, the order matters.

Strength Training Group 1
- Leg Extensions: 2 sets, 15 repetitions, page 105
- Lying Leg Curl: 2 sets, 12 repetitions, page 92
- Seated Leg Curl: 2 sets, 12 repetitions, page 95
- Wide Grip Front Pulldown: 2 sets, 15 repetitions, page 117
- Incline Dumbbell Press: 2 sets, 12 repetitions, page 128
- Pec Dec: 2 sets, 12 repetitions, page 106
- Front Dumbbell Raise: 2 sets, 12 repetitions, page 138
- Bent-Over Lateral Raise: 2 sets, 12 repetitions, page 131
- Close Grip Bench Press: 2 sets, 12 repetitions, page 120
- Dumbbell Concentration Curls: 2 sets, 12 repetitions, page 126
- Standing Calf Raise: 2 sets, 15 repetitions, page 96

Strength Training Group 2

- Hack Squat 2 sets: 15, then 12 repetitions, page 108
- Smith Machine Reverse Lunges: 2 sets: 15 repetitions each, page 104
- Leg Press: 2 sets, 15 repetitions each, page 89
- Seated Rows: 2 sets, 15 repetitions each, page 97
- Upright Rows: 2 sets, 12 repetitions each, page 144
- Chest Press Machine: 2 sets, 12 repetitions each, page 115
- Triceps Pressdown: 2 sets, 12 repetitions each, page 98
- Standing Barbell Curls: 2 sets 12 repetitions each, page 111
- Leg Press: 2 sets 15 repetitions each, page 89

Strength Training Group 3

- Smith Machine Squats: 2 sets, 15 repetitions each, page 103
- Leg Extensions: 2 sets, 15 repetitions each, page 105
- One Arm Dumbbell Rows: 2 sets, 15 repetitions each, page 127
- Good Mornings: 2 sets, 15 repetitions each, page 137
- Incline Dumbbell Press: 2 sets, 15 repetitions each, page 128
- Seated Dumbbell Press: 2 sets, 15 repetitions each, page 129
- Overhead Rope Extension: 2 sets, 15 repetitions each, page 101
- One Arm Preacher Curls: 2 sets, 15 repetitions each, page 123
- Standing Calf Raise: 2 sets, 15 repetitions each, page 96

Strength Training Group 4

- Leg Press: 2 sets, 15 repetitions each, page 89
- Barbell Squats: 2 sets, 15 repetitions each, page 112
- Lying Leg Curl: 2 sets, 10 repetitions each, page 92
- Bent-Over Dumbbell Rows: 2 sets, 15 repetitions each, page 136
- Assisted Push-Ups: 2 sets, 10 repetitions each, page 124
- One Arm Reverse-Grip Press Down: 2 sets, 15 repetitions each, page 99
- Bench Dips: 2 sets, 15 repetitions each, page 90
- Hammer Curls: 3 sets, 15 repetitions each, page 151
- Seated Calf Raise: 2 sets, 15 repetitions each, page 94

Cardiovascular Workout

Heart rate: 70 to 85% of maximum heart rate

Duration: 20 minutes

For the final stretch, I want you to use only once piece of equipment, six days a week. Do not choose one of the machines you used during the three-month workout program. Be sure to monitor you heart rate closely. Increase the intensity level every 1 minute.

Duration in minutes	Description	Maximum Heart Rate
1	warm-up	60%
1	medium intensity	65%
1	medium intensity	65%
1	high intensity	80%
1	high intensity	85%
1	recovery	55%
1	medium intensity	65%
1	medium intensity	65%
1	high intensity	80%
1	high intensity	85%
1	medium intensity	65%
1	recovery	55%
1	medium intensity	65%

Duration in minutes	Description	Maximum Heart Rate
1	medium intensity	65%
1	high intensity	80%
1	high intensity	80%
1	high intensity	85%
1	high intensity	85%
1	low intensity	60%
1	cool-down	55%

Post Workout Stretching

Heart Rate: 50% of maximum heart rate

Duration: 5 minutes

- Shoulder Blade Squeeze, page 164
- Rotator Cuff Stretch, page 164
- Sitting Twist, page 165
- External Rotation Stretch, page 165
- Ankle Reach, page 165
- Cat Stretch/Back Arch page 166
- Back Arch, page 166
- Half-Kneeling Shin Stretch, page 167

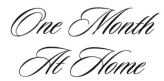

One Month At Home

Follow the same routines for the dynamic stretch, and post workout stretching as found in the gym version of the one month workout.

Warm-Up

Heart rate: 60% of your maximum heart rate

Duration: 5 minutes

You will need a jump rope for this warm-up. Jump rope in place, watching your footing as you go. Try and jump for five minutes without stopping. If you need to rest or get tripped up by the rope, stop briefly, and then resume your pace.

Abdominal Drills

Heart rate: 55% of maximum heart rate

Durations: 5 minutes

You will perform the same exercise as the gym workout except for some changes due to the lack of equipment. Again, choose two exercises from each group, upper, lower and obliques. Do two sets of 25 repetitions of each exercise. Complete all of the sets for that exercise before you proceed to the next. Cut down your rest period to only five seconds between exercises.

Abdominal Group 1 at Home
(Upper Abdominals)

- Butterfly Crunch, page 63
- Thigh Slide Crunch, page 64
- Basic Crunch, page 59

Abdominal Group 2 at Home (Obliques)

- Jackknife, page 76
- Twisting Crunch on the Physioball, page 73
- Cross Body Crunch, page 58

Abdominal Group 3 at Home
(Lower Abdominals)

- V-Ups, page 65
- Reverse Crunch, page 75
- Scissor Kick, page 66

Strength Training

Heart Rate Check: 65% of maximum heart rate

Duration: 20 minutes

Strength Training Group 1 at Home

- Dumbbell Squats: 2 sets, 20 repetitions each, page 141
- Alternating Dumbbell Lunges: 2 sets, 20 repetitions each, page 142
- Good Mornings: 2 sets, 20 repetitions each,

page 137

- Bent-Over Dumbbell Rows: 2 sets, 20 repetitions each, page 136
- Assisted Push-Ups: 2 sets, 15 repetitions each, page 124
- Seated Dumbbell Press: 2 sets: 12, then 10 repetitions, page 129
- Standing Dumbbell Kickback: 2 sets, 20 repetitions each, page 146
- Standing Dumbbell Curls: 2 sets, 20 repetitions each, page 140
- Standing One-Leg Calf Raise: 2 sets, 20 repetitions each, page 135

Strength Training Group 2

- Physioball Dumbbell Squats: 2 sets, 20 repetitions each, page 132
- Glute Lifts with Physioball: 2 sets 20 repetitions, page 149
- Stiff-Leg Dead Lifts: 2 sets, 20 repetitions each, page 133
- Flat Dumbbell Flyes: 2 sets, 15, 12 repetitions each, page 125
- Upright Rows: 2 sets, 15 repetitions each, page 144
- Chair Dips: 2 sets, 15 repetitions each, page 139

- Dumbbell Concentration: Curls 2 sets, 15 repetitions each, page 126
- Standing One-Leg Calf Raise: 2 sets, 20 repetitions each, page 135

Strength Training Group 3

- Dumbbell Lunges: 2 sets, 20 repetitions each, page 142
- Leg Lifts: 3 sets, 10 repetitions each, page 148
- Good Mornings: 2 sets, 20 repetitions each, page 137
- Assisted Push-ups: 2 sets, 15 repetitions each, page 124
- Side Lateral Raise: 2 sets, 20 repetitions each, page 147
- Front Dumbbell Raise: 2 sets, 20 repetitions each, page 138
- Seated Dumbbell Extension: 2 sets, 15 repetitions each, page 129
- Hammer Curls: 2 sets, 15 repetitions each, page 151
- Standing One-Leg Calf Raise: 2 sets, 20 repetitions each, page 135

Strength Training Group 4

- Physioball Dumbbell Squats: 2 sets, 20 repetitions each, page 132

- Dumbbell Lunges: 2 sets, 20 repetitions each, page 142
- Stiff-Leg Deadlift: 2 sets, 20 repetitions each, page 133
- Flat Bench Dumbbell: 2 sets, 20 repetitions each, page 110
- Bent-Over Lateral Raise: 2 sets, 20 repetitions each, page 131
- Upright Rows: 2 sets, 20 repetitions each, page 144
- Standing Dumbbell Kickback: 2 sets, 20 repetitions each, page 146
- Standing Dumbbell Curls: 2 sets, 15 repetitions each, page 140
- Standing One-Leg Calf Raise: 2 sets, 20 repetitions each, page 135

Aerobic Workout: High-intensity Interval Training

Heart rate: 75-80% of maximum heart rate

Durations: 20 minutes

At this point your endurance level is at full throttle. You should really be pushing yourself, and going all out with your cardiovascular session. You should be jumping rope for twenty minutes nonstop. Continue to monitor your heart rate. If you see that if is exceeding 80 percent of your maximum heart rate, slow down or stop.

If you do in-line skating or have a traditional bike, stick with one or the other for twenty minutes. No matter what you choose, be sure to check your heart rate so that you are training between 75 to 80 percent of your maximum heart rate. Continue to do your extra day of cardiovascular work, abdominal drills, and post workout stretch on Day 6 and 7.

Post Workout Stretching:

Heart rate: 50% of maximum heart rate

Duration: 5 Minutes

- Shoulder Blade Squeeze, page 164
- Rotator Cuff Stretch, page 164
- Sitting Twist, page 165
- External Rotation Stretch, page 165
- Ankle Reach, page 165
- Cat Stretch page 166
- Back Arch, page 166
- Half-Kneeling Shin Stretch, page 167

CONCLUSION:
Congratulations!

You've worked hard, and you've come a long way. Celebrate your accomplishments by taking a good hard look at yourself. Take a last set of photographs, and calculate your weight, body fat percentage, and body measurements. You should be pleased with the results.

The most important thing you can do for yourself at this point is relax. It is important physically as well as mentally. Get used to the whole new you, the ideals of married life, and beyond. About a week before the wedding, treat yourself to something truly special. Take some time to be by yourself and reflect on the work you've done. Now is a great time to do a little quiet meditation. Steal away to a quiet room, giving yourself fifteen to thirty minutes each evening. Think about all you've accomplished and what your new life will be like with your husband. Let go of all the planning and craziness for the wedding. Relax.

These suggestions can help:

- Buy candles and place them around the house, especially in your bedroom. Light them every night.
- Buy incense or an aroma therapy diffuser. Scent your favorite room in pleasant, herbal mist, or, take a nice, long, scented bath. Oils that are soothing are lavender and rosemary.
- Play soothing music like jazz, R&B, or old love songs.
- Take a low-impact yoga class, or buy an instructional video or book that focuses on the softer sides of yoga.

Speaking of the honeymoon, enjoy your romantic time with your new husband. Treat yourself to all of the foods that you wanted to eat while you were in *Bridal Bootcamp*™. Do not deprive yourself of the things that you like and crave. When you get back home, you'll get back to work.

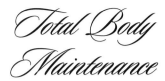

Total Body Maintenance

To maintain your bridal body from the honeymoon forward, we have to determine your caloric maintenance level. For example, Carol reached her goal before the wedding, weighing in at 130 pounds.

Let's see how she did overall.

Before	After:
Weight 160	Weight 135
Body fat 32%	Body fat 20%
Fat 51.2 lb.	Fat 27 lb.
Muscle 108.8 lb.	Muscle 108 lb.

Carol's final daily caloric maintenance level is 1781 calories. To maintain her current body composition, she will need to consume roughly 1800 per day.

It's always a good idea to strive to maintain a range between 5 to 10 pounds of your ideal weight. That way if you put on a few pounds, in less than one to two months you can take it right back off.

As always, if you want to maintain your hard body, you must continue to workout. If you just want to maintain your current physique, then continue to do your total body workouts at least three times per week.

Your wedding day is just the beginning of a whole new life for you. Now that you've completed *Bridal Bootcamp*™, you know that you can do anything once you set your mind to it. Bootcamp was hard, but you did it! I hope that you can take what you've learned here and keep up with the program, even after the honeymoon.

INDEX

A

Abdominal exercises
    at gym, 77–84
    at home, 55–76
    for one-month program, 258, 262
    for three-months program, 226–227, 232
    for six-months program, 193–194, 199–200
    time requirements for, 44
    tips for, 55
    warm-ups, 56
Abductor Machine, 113
Activity level multiplier, 18
Adductor Machine, 114
Aerobic workouts
    for one-month program, 154, 260–261, 264
    for three-months program, 154, 229–230, 234
    for six-months program, 154, 196, 202
    need for, 7–9
    target heart rate, 154, 196, 197
    time requirements for, 44
    tips for, 154
Alcohol consumption, 31
Alternating Dumbbell Lunges, 142
Alternating Front Dumbbell Raise, 145
American Shake, 36
Amino acids, 32
Ankle Reach Stretch, 165–166
Antioxidants, 41–42
Arm Circles, 50
Assisted Pull-Up Machine, 119
Assisted Push-Ups, 124
At-home program. See Home program

B

Back Arch Stretch, 166
Back: Folded Leaf Posture Stretch, 155
Back Reach Stretch, 160
Back Stretch, 158
Balanced foods, 26, 28, 171
Barbell Lunges, 109
Barbell Squats, 112
Basal energy expenditure (BEE), 17–18
Basal Metabolic Rate (BMR), 16
Basic Crunch, 59
Bench Dip, 90
Bent Knee Lunge, 161
Bent Leg Hip-Raise, 69
Bent-Over Dumbbell Rows, 136
Bent-Over Lateral Raise, 131

Berry Blend Smoothie, 34
Biceps Stretch, 156
Bicycle, 70, 202, 229, 234, 264
Binges, 31
Blood sugar levels, 24, 30
Body fat measurements, 19–22, 31, 169–170, 204, 206, 237, 266
Body measurements. See Girth measurements
Boredom, avoiding, 45
Brazilian Rain Smoothie, 35
Butterfly Crunch, 63
Byrd, Edward A., 19

C

Cable Crossover, 102
Cable Crunch with Rope, 81
Calcium, 38–41
Caloric maintenance level
    equations for, 16–20, 170, 206, 237
    maintaining, 30, 267
    understanding, 16
Calorie cutting, 172, 206, 237
Calorie requirements
    and metabolism, 16, 170
    and nutrition, 15–16
    determining, 17–20, 23–25, 170–171, 206, 237, 267
    monitoring, 172, 206
    see also Caloric maintenance level
Calves Stretch, 158
Camera, 14
Carbohydrates
    avoiding, 24–25
    daily requirements, 24, 171
    glycemic index, 205
    healthy choices, 25, 32, 205, 238
    importance of, 24, 205
Cardiovascular conditioning
    for one-month program, 154, 260–261, 264
    for three-months program, 154, 229–230, 234
    for six-months program, 154, 196, 202
    need for, 7–9
    target heart rate, 154, 196, 197
    time requirements for, 44
    tips for, 154
Cat Stretch/Back Arch, 166
Cellulite, 13
Chair Dip, 139
Chest Stretch, 155

Chiropractor consultation, 11
Cleanser Smoothie, 35
Close Grip Bench Press, 120
Clothing for exercising, 12
Complete Book of Food Counts, The, 29, 170
Cool-down stretches
    for one-month program, 164–167
    for three-months program, 159–163
    for six-months program, 155–158
    time requirements for, 44
Cow's milk, 32
Cravings, 26–27
Cross Body-Crunch, 58
Cross Over Split-Leg Crunch, 62

D

Daily caloric maintenance level. See Caloric maintenance level
Daily calorie needs. See Calorie requirements
Decline-Bench Twisting Crunch, 78
Dessert Surprise, 37
Diet program, 7–9, 11, 15–37. See also Meal plans
Doctor consultation, 11
Double Crunch, 61
Dumbbell Concentration Curls, 126
Dumbbell Shrugs, 152
Dumbbell Squats, 141
Dynamic stretching
    for one-month program, 257–258
    for three-months program, 226
    for six-months program, 193, 199

E

Eating habits, 16, 26, 30. See also Meal plans
Elliptical climber, 229, 230
Energy Balanced Diet, The, 26
Energy needs, 16–22, 28, 30, 236
Equipment needs, 11–14
Exercise program
    abdominal exercises, 57–84
    before starting, 11–14
    equipment for, 11–14
    for one-month program, 257–264
    for three-months program, 225–235
    for six-months program, 191–203
    location of, 11, 45
    strength training exercises, 85–153
    stretches, 154–167, 198, 202–203
    success of, 7–9
    warm-ups, 45–54
    see also specific exercises
External Rotation Stretch, 165
Extreme foods, 26, 31

F

Fats, 25, 154, 171
Fetal Position Stretch, 158
Fiber, 25, 205
Figure-Four Crunch, 72
Fitness program. See Exercise program; Nutrition program
Flat Dumbbell Flyes, 125
Flat Dumbbell Press, 110
Flexibility, 154
Flutter Kick, 47
Food diary, 31, 169, 172. See also Journal
Food groups, 28, 171
Food scale, 14
Foods
    balanced foods, 26, 28, 171
    effects of, 26
    extreme foods, 26, 31
    glycemic foods, 205, 238
    trigger foods, 15, 26, 31
    see also Meal plans
Front Dumbbell Raise, 138
Fruits, 205, 238

G

Girth measurements, 14, 169, 204, 237, 266
Glute Lifts with Physioball, 149
Glutes Stretch, 157–158
Glycemic carbohydrates, 238
Glycemic index, 205
Goat's milk, 32
Gold's Gym, 45
Good Mornings, 137
Gotein, 32
Green leafy vegetables, 28
Grocery shopping tips, 31
Gym workout
    abdominal exercises, 77–84
    for one-month program, 257–261
    for three-months program, 226–231
    for six-months program, 193–198
    strength training exercises, 85–129

H

Hack Squat, 108
Half-Kneeling Shin Stretch, 167
Hammer Curls, 151
Hamstrings Stretch, 157, 161–162
Hands over Head Crunch, 71
Hanging Knee Raise to the Side, 83
Hanging Run-in-Place, 80
Harris-Benedict equation, 16–18
Head Lean Stretch, 159
Health food stores, 32

Heart rate
    determining, 191–192
    monitor for, 12, 192
    target heart rate, 55, 85, 154, 196, 197
Herbal supplements, 39–40
High-intensity interval training
    for one-month program, 264
    for three-months program, 234
    for six-months program, 196–197
Hip Stretch, 157–158
Hip Swing, 54
Hip Thrust, 74
Home program
    abdominal exercises, 55–76
    for one-month program, 262–264
    for three-months program, 232–235
    for six-months program, 199–205
    strength training exercises, 130–153

I

In-line skates, 202, 234, 264
Incline Dumbbell Press, 128
Iso-Pure Zero Carbs, 32

J

Java Junkies Shake, 36
Jaw Tuck Stretch, 160
Journal, 13–14, 16, 20, 22, 31, 169–170, 172,
    204, 237, 266
Jump rope, 202, 234, 264
Jumping Jacks, 49
Jumping Squats, 54

K

Kick-Out with Jumping Jacks, 53

L

Label-reading, 31
Lateral Stride Stretch, 162
Lean body mass, 24
Lean muscle mass, 20–22, 170
Leg Extensions, 105
Leg Lifts, 148
Leg Press, 89
Leg Press Calf Raise, 93
Lower Back Stretch, 158
Lying Leg Curl, 92
Lying Triceps Barbell Extension, 118

M

Machine Crunch, 82
Magnesium, 38–41
Maintaining weight loss, 267
Meal plans
    following, 171
    for one-month program, 238–256
    for three-months program, 207–224
    for six-months program, 172–190
    meal replacement guide, 32
    meal-skipping, 30
    meals per day, 30
    preparation for, 27, 31
    rules for, 30–31
    sets of, 16, 29–30
    understanding, 171
Measurements, recording, 14, 169–170,
    204, 237, 266
Measuring cups, 14
Measuring tape, 14
Measuring tips, 14
Medical Research Institute, 19
Medicine Ball Rotations, 51–52
Metabolism, 16, 170
Milk, 32
Minerals, 38–43
Mountain Climbers, 47
Multivitamins, 38–43
Muscle loss, 21–22, 170, 206
Muscle mass, 20–22, 170
Muscle tissue, 19–22, 154, 170, 196

N

Natural foods, 15
Neck Stretch, 156
Netzer, Corrine T., 29, 170
Notebook, 13. See also Journal
Nutrient ratio, 29, 171
Nutrients, 38–43
Nutrition program, 15–37. See also Meal plans
Nutritional needs, 7–8, 15–16

O

Oblique Crunch, 60
One Arm Dumbbell Rows, 127
One Arm Preacher Dumbbell Curls, 123
One Arm Reverse-Grip Press Down, 99
One-month program
    abdominal exercises, 258, 262
    aerobic workout, 260–261, 264
    at gym, 257–261
    at home, 262–264
    meal plan for, 238–256

strength training, 258–260, 262–264
stretches, 164–167, 257–258, 261, 264
warm-ups, 53–54, 257, 262
workout for, 257–264
Overhead Lateral Raise, 143
Overhead Rope Extension, 101

P

Peanut Butter Paradise Shake, 33
Pec Dec, 106
Photographs, 14, 204, 236–237, 266
Physioball Dumbbell Squats, 132
Physioball One Arm Dumbbell Extensions, 134
Physioball Push-Ups, 150
Plank Posture with Downward Facing Dog, 51
Post-workout stretching
    for one-month program, 261, 264
    for three-months program, 235
    for six-months program, 198, 202–203
    time requirements for, 44
Preacher Curls, 107
Prisoner Squats, 50
Processed foods, 15
Protein, 23–24, 28, 32, 171
Protein bars, 32
Protein shakes, 32–36

Q

Quadriceps Stretch, 157

R

Rear Deltoid Flyes, 91
Recipes, 33–37
Record-keeping, 13–14, 16, 20, 22, 31, 169–170,
    172, 204, 237, 266
Relaxation, 203, 235, 266
Resting Metabolic Rate (RMR), 16
Reverse Crunch, 75
Reverse Crunch on Incline Board, 84
Reverse Crunch with Physioball, 68
Rosenthal, Joshua, 26
Rotator Cuff Stretch, 164
Running, 202, 229

S

Salty food cravings, 27
Scale, 13, 14, 31
Scissors Kick, 66
Seated Cable Rows, 97
Seated Calf Raise Machine, 94

Seated Dumbbell Press, 129
Seated Leg Curls, 95
Seated Machine Press, 115
Seated Overhead Dumbbell Extension, 153
Seven-day meal plan
    for one-month program, 238–256
    for three-months program, 207–224
    for six-months program, 172–190
    see also Meal plans
Shakes, 32–36
Shoes for exercising, 12
Shopping tips, 31
Shoulder Blade Squeeze, 164
Shoulder Press Machine, 116
Shoulder Stretch, 155
Side Bend, 67
Side Jackknife, 76
Side Lateral Dumbbell Raise, 147
Single-Leg Squat Touchdown, 50
Sitting Twist Stretch, 165
Six-months program
    abdominal exercises, 193–194, 199–200
    aerobic workouts, 154, 196, 202
    at gym, 193–198
    at home, 199–205
    meal plan for, 172–190
    strength training, 194–195, 200–201
    stretches, 155–158, 193, 198, 199, 202–203
    warm-ups, 47–49, 193, 199
    workout for, 191–203
Skinfold caliper, 19–20, 169
Slim Guide Caliper, 19
Smith Machine Reverse Lunges, 104
Smith Machine Squats, 103
Smoothies, 32, 34–35
Snacks, 32–37
Spine Rotation Stretch, 162
Squat Stretch, 157–158
Squat Thrusts, 48
Stair climber, 202, 229, 230
Standing Barbell Curls, 111
Standing Calf Raise, 96
Standing Dumbbell Curls, 140
Standing Dumbbell Kickback, 146
Standing Leg Curl, 121
Standing One Leg Calf Raise, 135
Starburst, 53
Starting program, 11–14
Static stretching, 154
Stiff-Leg Deadlift, 133
Strawberry Fields Smoothie, 34
Strawberry Granola Fruit Parfait, 37

Strength training
    at gym, 85–129
    at home, 130–153
    for one-month program, 258–260, 262–264
    for three-months program, 227–228, 233–234
    for six-months program, 194–195, 200–201
    misconceptions, 122
    need for, 7–9
    sets, 85–86
    time requirements for, 44
    tips for, 85–86
Stretches
    for one-month program, 164–167, 257–258, 261, 264
    for three-months program, 159–163, 231, 236
    for six-months program, 155–158, 193, 198, 199, 202–203
    post-workout stretching, 154–167, 198, 202–203, 235, 261, 264
    time requirements for, 44
Success of program, 7–9
Supplements, 7–8, 38–43
Sweet cravings, 27
Sweet vegetables, 28

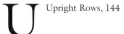

Tape measure, 14
Thigh-Slide Crunch, 64
Three-months program
    abdominal exercises, 226–227, 232
    aerobic workout, 154, 229–230, 234
    at gym, 225–231
    at home, 232–235
    meal plan for, 207–224
    strength training, 227–228, 233–234
    stretches, 159–163, 226, 231
    warm-ups, 50–52, 226
    workout for, 225–235
Toxins, flushing, 13, 15, 28
Treadmill, 197, 202, 229
Triceps Pressdown, 98
Triceps Stretch, 156
Trigger foods, 15, 26, 31
Twisting Crunch on the Physioball, 73
Two Arm High Cable Curl, 100

U Upright Rows, 144

V V-Ups, 65
Vegetables, 28, 205, 238
Vegetarian protein sources, 23
Vertical-Bench Leg Raise, 79
Vitamins, 38–43

W Walking, 202, 229
Walking Lunge with Twist, 48
Wall Stretch, 159, 163
Warm-ups
    for one-month program, 53–54, 257, 262
    for three-months program, 50–52, 226
    for six-months program, 47–49, 193, 199
    time requirements for, 44
    tips for, 45–46
Water consumption
    avoiding during meals, 29
    daily requirements, 28–29
    during exercise, 28–29
    for flushing toxins, 13, 15, 28
    importance of, 15, 28–29, 31
    water method, 28–29
Weighing in, 13, 31, 169–170, 204, 237, 266
Weight lifting tips, 85–86. See also Strength training
Weight loss
    goal for, 15–16, 21–22, 169–170
    maintaining, 267
    per week, 19, 21–22, 170, 206
    tips for, 30–31
Weight scale, 13, 31
Whey proteins, 32
Whole grains, 28, 205, 238
Wide Grip Front Pulldown, 117
Workouts
    for one-month program, 257–264
    for three-months program, 225–235
    for six-months program, 191–203
    see also Exercise program
Wrist Stretch, 160–161

Y Yoga Cobra Posture, 56
Yoga Stretches, 51